Anton Chekhov famously joked that medicine was his wife and literature his mistress, so it's tempting to say the same for any doctor who moonlights as a writer. But I'm pretty sure Chekhov said this with his tongue firmly in his cheek, for certainly a man obsessed with human complexity did not believe his two passions could be so cleanly divided.

Ron Lands writes beautiful stories about the messiness of sickness, death, loss, confusion, and compassion. In his work, his two worlds of doctor and writer seamlessly overlap. Most of the men and women who populate these stories are facing the end—either their own, or someone else's— and the medical, practical, emotional, and spiritual complexities that develop in the final hours and days intertwine to create moving and memorable conflicts between, and within, the characters.

These stories take place in the homes, doctor's offices, and hospital rooms of a small Tennessee town, where doctors intimately know their patients, and patients exist in a generational no-mans' land between house calls and contemporary medicine. Lands' ability to explore their humanity as his characters navigate the unfamiliar makes these stories shimmer. Beautifully rendered sentence after sentence, *The Long Way Home* is the work of an expert in his fields.

—Susan Perabo, author of *The Fall of Lisa Bellow*

OTHER BOOKS BY RON LANDS

Final Path, Finishing Line Press, Spring 2020

A Gathering of Friends, Main Street Rag,
   Forthcoming, 2021

APPALACHIAN SERIES

BOTTOM DOG PRESS

THE LONG WAY HOME

RON LANDS

APPALACHIAN SERIES
BOTTOM DOG PRESS
HURON, OHIO 44839

ISBN: 978-1-947504-12-7
Bottom Dog Press, Inc.
PO Box 425, Huron, OH 44839
Lsmithdog@aol.com
http://smithdocs.net

CREDITS:
General Editor: Larry Smith
Layout and Cover Design: Susanna Sharp-Schwacke
Cover Image: Coker/ Alamy Stock Photo

ACKNOWLEDGMENTS:

"The Rebellion of Katie Lane," *The Fourth River*; "Fogs of
August," *Wind*; "The Diving Bell," *Washington Square*; "Ashes
to Ashes," *Breathing the Same Air, Anthology of East Tennessee Writers*; "This Old House," *The Portland Literary Review*;
"Span of Life," *descant*; "Runaway," *New Millennium Writings*; "What Noma Meant to Say," *Floyd County Moonshine*;
"The Veil," *The Distillery* and *Surreal South*; "The Healer,"
Nassau Review; "Heart Sounds," *The Big Muddy*; "The Long
Way Home," *RiverSedge*; "Reflections," *New Millenniu Writings*; "Avy's Place," *Branchwood Journal*; "Charlie Benson Sees
the Ocean," *Conte, Journal of Narrative Writing*.

These stories are for my patients who still give me
a reason to write, and my wife, Jackie, who gives me space
to do it.

TABLE OF CONTENTS

THE REBELLION OF KATIE LANE 7

THE FOGS OF AUGUST 17

THE DIVING BELL 29

ASHES TO ASHES 37

THIS OLD HOUSE 45

SPAN OF LIFE 56

RUNAWAY 65

WHAT NOMA MEANT TO SAY 75

THE VEIL 83

THE HEALER 92

HEART SOUNDS 109

THE LONG WAY HOME 123

REFLECTIONS 131

AVY'S PLACE 143

CHARLIE BENSON SEES THE OCEAN 152

ABOUT THE AUTHOR 165

THE REBELLION OF KATIE LANE

For the first seventeen years of our lives we were friends, not a couple, just next-door neighbors in one-story white-frame dwellings left over from when the coal companies provided housing for their employees. Ours were the last two on a dead-end street that was marked on the far side by Black's Creek, and on the other by a cracked, concrete sidewalk that rolled and swelled past our tiny yards then stopped in a vacant lot as if it had reached the end of the world.

From the outside, my house looked the same as Billy's: tiny windows with soot-stained white paint chipping off the sills, a little porch that swayed in the middle and gave the false impression of a smile, a gravel driveway just big enough for one car, and a bare lightbulb by the front door.

On the inside, we couldn't have been more different. My mom wore a homemade cotton dress, sat all day at our upright piano, and played slow mournful hymns. Billy's mom came home from her job waitressing at the Peggy Ann Truck Stop, put on cutoff blue jeans, a "See Rock City" tee shirt, and mowed their yard in her bare feet. My dad was somber, strict, given to dissecting the King James Version at the supper table long after Mom and I had brushed our hair, put on our nightgowns, and gone to bed. Billy didn't know his dad.

On Sundays, my dad drove us so far back into the mountains that the gravel roads turned to dirt, to a renovated house with a sign out front that said, "Church of the Mighty God." Inside, we sat on hard benches while an old man yelled a sermon at us. Billy's mom took him to the Peggy Ann, where I imagined him lounging all day immersed in the thick, heavy smell of fried onions and hamburgers.

"What do you do while you wait?" I asked.

"Read," he said showing me a Zane Grey Western all dog-eared and yellow. "The truckers leave these in a box. They take one and leave the one they just read. You can read 'em, too. I'll bring you one."

I wasn't old enough then to be surprised that Billy could enjoy a novel about the wild west or that he thought a seven-year-old girl would, too.

By the time I was in junior high, I looked like a miniature version of my mother, with long hair and dresses that reached to my wrists, ankles, and throat. My class-mates laughed at me, told me I looked like I had stepped off a covered wagon in the middle of the prairie, just like on *Gunsmoke* or *Bonanza*. It was years before I knew what they were talking about. We didn't have a television. Dad had convictions against it, saw it as a tool of the Antichrist, a sign of the End Times.

When I asked Mom why we had to be so different, she sent me to Dad.

"It's an outward sign of an inward change," he said, as if I had ever known another way. Then he made me car-ry a New Testament in my book satchel to make me even more different. "Read it when the others are on the play-ground," he said. "It'll set you apart. They won't bother you with worldly things."

When I was a senior, I found my mother's 1950 high school yearbook where she hid it in the back of her closet. There was a picture of her wearing a cheerleading outfit, a black skirt just above her knees, white bobby socks, saddle oxfords, and a sweater with a monogram on the front of a bearded little coal miner with a shovel over his shoulder and Oak Grove Miners emblazoned on a banner waving over his head.

There was Dad's graduation picture with him wearing a tuxedo coat and a bow tie. His eyes twinkled. He had a mischievous smile. He didn't look like the man I'd heard testify about how he'd answered an evangelist's invitation at a tent revival and gave up his sinful earthly life in hopes of a heavenly eternal one. "I wasn't a murderer or a thief," he said. "But I realized that night that I carried the sin of Adam, that I was drifting down a river toward a lake of fire where I'd burn for eternity if I didn't change. I knelt at that knotty pine altar and begged God to save me. When I stood up, I was washed in the blood of Jesus, a brand-new man." Mom and Dad had changed so much, they were even different from themselves.

Because of their inward change, I was seventeen and had never attended a football game, hadn't been to a movie, and hadn't had a date, except for when Billy and I sat on our front porch in the arc of the bare lightbulb and talked, just like when we were little. I don't know why he kept coming over. I suspected that he felt sorry for me. I wonder, now, if he was lonely, too. I know I was enthralled by him, his theories, his ability to reason things out. I would listen to him for as long as he would talk.

When we were young, his questions were innocent, playful. "If you ate one of these oatmeal cookies every day, how many days would it take for you to gain one pound?" I never knew the answer. He always had a lengthy explanation.

As we got older, his questions were deeper, more cynical. "You know God only has one eye, don't you?"

"Don't joke that way. It's sacrilegious." I said it loud, so Dad would hear me if he happened to be eavesdropping.

"I'm not joking," he continued. "It says so in that song your momma plays."

I didn't know he listened to her, didn't realize he knew the words. I couldn't place the song myself.

"The one that says, 'His eye is on the sparrow and I know He watches me.'" He grinned. "His *eye*, not His *eyes*," he said mimicking the way Dad would take one pivotal word, one precise letter, one subtle change of tense or time, and create another requirement for a disciplined Christian life. "Singular, not plural," he continued. He pretended to glare at me, the way Dad clinched his arguments. Then he stared at the moon until a cloud floated in front of it. "Look," he said. "God blinked first."

I cringed and waited for Dad to explode through the screen door. When he didn't, I waited for a lightning bolt that would turn us both into Peggy Ann French fries.

Billy had the highest grades in our graduating class, so he had to give the valedictory speech. His was not one of those boring talks I've heard a dozen times since, about getting involved or making a difference. He talked like he did on my porch, confident, challenging, full of ambition, but he talked about things I had never heard, about aiming high, breaking free, exploring life.

Billy's mom sat on the front row wearing a backless, yellow sundress, mouthing the words with him. My parents sat in the back, two frowning silhouettes with their hands clasped in their laps as if they were trying to avoid joining the applause when Billy finished his speech.

After the ceremony was over and most of the Class of 1968 postponed adulthood for twenty-four more hours with an all-night dance in the Presbyterian Church basement, I rode home in the backseat of Dad's Chevrolet, remembering Billy's speech, thinking about all he said, and wondering what he meant.

*   *   *

The week after graduation, we sat down to supper with the windows open because the house was already hot. I was feeling more trapped than usual, imagining myself sitting at this table as a feeble old woman listening to Dad say grace.

"Bless this food to the nourishment of our bodies..." Dad said. Outside, a car engine revved, screamed for a few seconds, then cracked and backfired down to an irregular, rough idle.

Ignoring the racket, Dad rested his elbows on the table, and leaned toward me while Mom filled his plate. He combined our meals with Bible study, teaching by illustrating others' failures. "It's about what I'd expect," he said. He always assumed we knew who and what he was talking about, never gave any preamble as to what the moral of his story was going to be. "Carrie's mother had a reputation when your mom and I were in high school."

Carrie was a cheerleader, one of the many girls in my class that I envied from a distance. Her mother's picture was in Mom's yearbook too—Homecoming Queen, 1950. Carrie looked like her mother did: glamorous smile, blond hair, pretty figure.

"Doc Haskins wouldn't do it for her," Dad said, quirking his eyebrows to let us know such transparent claims didn't fool him.

Wouldn't do what, I wondered. I knew Carrie was getting married in a couple of weeks, but that wasn't unusual in Oak Grove. The majority of my class, even the ones with good grades, had no plans beyond getting a job and starting a family.

Dad cut viciously at the hamburger patty Mom served like steak. "Course he same *as* did it in God's eyes, if he'd told her where to get it done." He pursed his lips the way Billy enjoyed mimicking him, pulled himself straight, and pointed his fork at me for emphasis, like that would clarify any lingering questions I had. He nodded at Mom as if to give her permission to speak.

She didn't answer. She had long ago abandoned any pretense of being anything more than a prop at these evening sermons. She rearranged her mashed potatoes, smushed the middle gently with the bottom of her spoon, then ladled gravy into the little pool.

I wondered where he'd heard all this. Carrie's mom owned the beauty parlor where women exchanged gossip, but Mom didn't go there. Dad was a sewing machine fixer at the hosiery mill, but I couldn't picture him gossiping with the women who sewed.

He leaned toward me as if he was about to share a secret. "There's something a boy wants from a girl that she can only give away once. A teenage boy is like a dog. No thinking, just reacting to his base instincts."

Mom cut one side out of her mashed potato pond and watched the gravy dribble over the soft white bank. The motor revved, this time to a high whine, and it held there for almost a minute. Dad stopped in the middle of a quotation from somewhere in the Book of Revelations and glared at me as if the racket was my fault. Mom stood, wiped her hands on her apron, and walked to the front door.

I followed and looked over her shoulder. Billy had parked a candy-apple red Mustang in his drive and was listening studiously as the motor grumbled and growled. He had told me his mom had borrowed money to buy him a car from a trucker who was leaving for Vietnam.

I ran down the back steps, across our yard while Dad stood on our porch with his arms folded. Mom wiped her hands slowly over and over on her apron. I circled the car. The rear end was a good four inches higher than the front, and wide racing tires stuck out from under the fenders. The powerful motor made the car tremble like something alive. I recognized Creedence Clearwater Revival's "Bad Moon Rising" blaring from the rear speakers. I had listened to it late at night on WOAK with my ear close to a small plastic transistor radio that Billy had given me.

"It looks...like it's getting ready to jump on something," I said.

Billy stepped back, studied for a minute, and grinned at me. "It definitely has a feral attitude," he said. He loved to use words I didn't know. "You wanta go for a spin?"

I walked back to the porch. I looked at Dad. "Can I go?" I asked.

"Hell is real, Katie," Dad said. "Eternity is a long, long time."

I looked at Mom, who bit her lip and looked away.

I walked between them, into the house. Behind me, I heard the motor settle down as Billy engaged the clutch and backed into the street. When I looked out my bedroom window, he was gone.

I spent that summer hoping Billy would kidnap me and take me where the two of us would live happily ever after. I sat on our porch, watched him come and go while avoiding eye contact with me, and imagined sitting on a pillow between the Mustang's bucket seats so I could lean on Billy's shoulder while we raced the straight stretch of highway between Oak Grove and Blue Springs with the gauges glowing on the dashboard, the engine whining, and the wind whipping through the open windows.

I sat through Dad's supper sermons, wearing my long sleeves and long skirts during the hottest days, while I imagined wading with Billy in the shallow water out at Moonlight Bay. I sat through Sunday services at the Church of the Mighty God, picturing Billy and me lying on a blanket on a Tennessee River bank looking straight up at the sky, him identifying cloud formations, and me fighting the sensation that I was falling up.

It was mid-August when he came to see me again. He sat in the car, staring through the windshield into space for a full minute after he turned off the motor. I waited on the porch. He finally came over, sat down on the top step beside me, and leaned against the railing. We both watched the sky, avoiding looking at each other. It was clear, early evening, so I could still see the Smoky Mountains with their tops wearing small clouds like little party hats.

"I'm leaving tomorrow," he said. His voice was subdued, almost a whisper, as if he had just confessed to drowning a sack of kittens. "I'm going to college." He didn't look at me. "They gave me a scholarship to UT."

I had to struggle to think and breathe at the same time. Scholarship? He hadn't told me…anything. Why couldn't he just get a job? Why not join the Navy? Why did he have to go to the one place where small-town people don't come back from?

"What about me?" My voice croaked.

He glanced at me for a split second, then he looked toward the mountains like a thousand other times when I thought he was only looking at the horizon, not imagining what was on the other side.

"There's more scholarships," he said, as if he was a wise grown-up dispensing advice to a naïve youngster, as if he didn't know my parents would never let me go to college even if they did have the money. "You've got good grades."

"Stay here," I said. I knew Dad was probably listening on the other side of the door. I didn't care. I moved close, knelt with my knees between Billy's feet, took his face in my hands, turned him to where I could see his eyes. "You can work at the hosiery mill…" I felt his face harden forcing him to look at me again. "If you love me, you won't go," I said. I wanted those words back the minute I heard them come out of my mouth. Billy took my wrists, lifted my hands away without looking at me and walked back to his car. I couldn't stop myself from saying them again and again.

Dr. Haskins had my medical file on his knees, fumbled with the two or three pages that gave the details of when my mother had me, the flow chart of all my vaccinations, the one or two visits when I came in for stomach flu or an earache. His wire-rimmed glasses pinched the tip end of his nose where they didn't get in the way of his eyes. His knobby hands were gnarled with arthritis, as ugly as any farmer's, only without the calluses or the dirt ground into the seams. I wondered how he sewed up cuts, wondered if his hands were why he quit delivering babies.

He smiled, as if he was proud. "So you're going to college," he said.

Billy was the first person who ever mentioned college to me, and I didn't think he meant it. Doc said it as if he assumed I would better myself. It made me feel a little easier about what I wanted to ask.

"I'm not here for a physical," I said.

"Really?" Doc said, as if he was surprised. "Is something wrong?" He didn't seem the least impatient or in a hurry, but I felt like I was wasting his time.

I told him about Billy and me—how since he left, I felt like I had no way out, as if my horizons stopped at the sidewalk at the end of our street.

"You're pregnant?" he asked. He pinched the bridge of his nose, squinched his eyes tight, as if he dreaded the answer.

"No," I said. My face burned. Not even my mother had asked me a question so private. "I don't need your help…that way."

Doc rearranged the wrinkles furrowed into his face from sad to tired and studied me, as if he was noticing for the first time, my dress, my hair, my lack of jewelry or makeup—as if he had only just remembered my parents.

"How can I help?"

Cicadas blended their singing with the low, thrumming rhythm of the table fan that turned slowly back and forth trying to stir the hot August air around my bed. I stood in front of my mirror, adjusted the baseball cap that fit loosely after I hacked off most of my hair. I buttoned the flannel shirt and tightened the jeans Doc's wife had scrounged out of their church's poor closet.

I opened a brown grocery sack that held a change of clothes, an envelope with fifty dollars and a one-way bus ticket to a small town in Kentucky. I fingered the note with a name and phone number of a friend of Doc Haskins or his wife, someone I didn't know, someone who would help me get started in a college where the students worked for their tuition, a place where I wouldn't need to tell my parents until it was too late for them to interfere.

Outside, the wind stirred the leaves in the oak tree. The air thickened with the smell of rain not yet fallen. I tried to imagine Billy at that big university in Knoxville, wondering if he was lonesome, afraid, whether he ever thought of me. I wondered when it was I quit just knowing him and started loving him.

I looked toward where I imagined him to be, but all I saw was a few stars scattered like shards of broken glass in an oil-black sky, dark enough that on other nights I would have worried about eternity. The cold full moon glared down at me like God's unblinking eye.

I glared right back.

THE FOGS OF AUGUST

The noise in the woods around my cabin blurred the sound of the telephone ringing. I listened to the creaking and croaking of tree frogs, crickets, and the wail of a small animal lost to a larger one in nature's food chain. I let the phone sound off a few more times before I answered.

"Tommy?" Mom said. "Are you all right?" Mom's the only one who will let it ring until I decide to pick it up.

I told her I was fine.

While she talked, I looked down at the house where I grew up. I live in a cabin on a corner of the farm, up on a bluff, out of the way. I like it here, and can see the whole valley from my bedroom window. Some nights, when I can't separate now from then, here from there, present from past, I sit here all night, remembering.

When a young man, my dad mounted a floodlight on the front of the barn that kept the whole yard bright all night. He told my brother and me that it kept away tigers. He loved for us to tell him there weren't any around here, so he could say "See? It's working." Tonight, the barn was dark.

I asked Mom why the light wasn't on.

"I was trying to put Ewell to bed," she said. "If he sees a light, he thinks it means he needs to get up."

He used to be a big man, full of grand ideas and sage advice, known for his generosity, his honesty and his ability to scratch a living out of Appalachian dirt. He's not any of that now. Once Mom called to tell me that he had her trapped upstairs. "He's sitting in a dining room chair on the bottom landing," she said. "He has his walking cane, and he pokes it at me like a sword every time I move." Those were hard times. That was when he spent his nights reliving his experience at Normandy—scared, wet, and wounded—and his days searching the house for one of the many lovers he was convinced my mother had taken.

Now, he follows Mom around, holding onto her shoulder, and shuffling his feet, his body tilted forward, his mouth fixed into a mask-like frown. She lets him work puzzles with the big pieces.

I asked if she wanted me to come down there.

"No," she said. "I just wanted to remind you that you are driving us to church in the morning."

Mom never had a reason to drive when Dad was healthy. She tried to take herself places after he had to quit. She could keep out of the way of oncoming traffic, but she couldn't remember the little things, like keeping gas in the tank. Both times she ran out, I had to carry a can of gas to the middle of town, in front of the post office, in front of all the people in Oak Grove who knew about me. They knew that I went to the war and came back different, knew I didn't like to be in crowds, knew I didn't like to talk. They were people who thought they knew me but would fear me if they knew what I knew about myself. I hated their prying eyes.

The second time I asked her if the gas gauge was broken.

"Yes," she said, "I think it is." She bit down hard on her lip, like she was making it quit talking. When we got home, she stood with her arms folded, watching me while I took the dashboard apart, checking the wiring and the needle gauge. I was contemplating whether or not to pull the gas tank and check the float valve when I realized that the car was fine. Dad had monitored everything for her for so long that she didn't know if her tank was half full or half empty.

I told her I didn't think I could fix it.

"Me neither," she said. "We just have to deal with it."

I've been driving them everywhere, ever since.

This Sunday was homecoming or something. People from everywhere were going to be there; people who grew up and moved away, people who grew up and stayed. Anyone with a history that trekked through the Asbury Methodist Church of Oak Grove was invited. It would be good for me, Mom said, to renew some of my old ties, to come down off the hill and act like a human being for one day.

I don't get a lot out of church anymore. It makes me feel cheap, mean, and dirty. It was only after I agreed to go that she mentioned that my brother was going to be there, too. He makes me feel the same way.

It's not his fault. I'm the one who thought anything more than a passing grade in school was wasted effort. I'm the one who was an all-state athlete in three sports, and never planned to go to college. I'm the one whose younger brother was the valedictorian of his graduating class. I'm the one who joined the Army on his birthday and who moved away, grew up, and came back, but never came home. I'm the prodigal son of the most upright parents in New Hope valley.

I smoked a whole pack of unfiltered Lucky Strikes while the moon stalked the stars across the sky. I still had the phone in my lap when the sun came up and chased them away. I went to the bathroom and splashed cold water on my face, looked in the mirror at my reflection. For a minute, I didn't know which one of us was real.

The headlamps on my truck could barely penetrate the fog that had rolled off the Tennessee River and was only starting to burn away by ten a.m. "Gonna be a white Christmas," Mom said. She used to predict winter storms by counting the fogs in August. She'd already marked this one on the calendar hanging in her kitchen.

I didn't answer. Dad kept leaning over more and more on my shoulder, so I had to drive using only my left hand. With my rebuilt left foot and a stiff left knee, I have to concentrate to work the clutch and change gears.

I wound around the country road, following the river to the edge of town. I pulled my truck into the parking lot of a small white church with a picture book steeple on it. I noticed the gun-metal grey Mercedes coupe parked alone, away from all the other trucks and cars. Even Dennis's car was better than the rest of us. I wondered if he brought his little blonde wife with the Chiclet teeth; then I remembered that Mom told me she had divorced him.

I parked under the big oak tree that was a sapling when the original congregation met in a brush arbor in the early 1800s. I rolled Dad in his wheelchair across the gravel parking lot, and up the ramp he had helped build for other invalids decades ago.

Dennis was already inside, shaking hands with everybody, smiling and talking, acting like he was the host, welcoming all the visitors. He'd remember everyone's name or fake it so well they would think he did. I was never that way.

His shiny penny loafers, button-down collars and starched khaki pants camouflaged his past, hid the fact that he once bailed hay, cut tobacco, and shoveled manure out of the same cold wet barn as I did.

I wished I had thought to shave, to clip my fingernails. I tucked my nose into my shirt sleeve, while nobody was looking. I smelled like an ash tray. I ran my fingers through my hair.

It didn't matter. Whatever common ground we once shared had long ago eroded, leaving us nothing solid to stand on. I got my third purple heart while he was pledging some fraternity. They discharged me from Walter Reed the summer he graduated from law school. I am who I am. He's a partner with the biggest law firm in Knoxville.

Dennis waved at me as I rolled Dad to his pew and parked him in the aisle. He tried to separate himself from a vaguely familiar old couple who were hanging onto his arm. I'm a little sensitive about it, I guess, but they seemed to keep eyeing me from time to time, probably telling him how they had predicted he would amount to something big. Country people are proud when one of their small-town, farm boys make good.

He waved at me again, inviting me to join them. I mimed back at him that I needed to go to the bathroom. I walked to the back of the sanctuary and down the stairs to the basement. It was cool, damp. I looked in the tiny Sunday school rooms, remembered when Dennis and I sat on those tiny little chairs, wearing our burr haircuts, homemade shirts, and listened to "Miss Loretta" tell us about Abraham taking his son up the mountain to offer him as a sacrifice, just because a powerful Somebody told him to.

I glanced at the bookshelf tacked on the wall in the hallway, sagging from neglect, not from the weight of the dozen or so paperback books. They were the same stories, missionaries who had suffered and died trying to convert the heathen, God's messengers who were eaten by cannibals while trying to spread the gospel all over the world. I had read them all.

It got quiet upstairs. I heard a muffled invocation, followed by brogans scraping on hardwood, imagined the rustle of pages turning in hymnals. I walked up to the landing where I could see. Dennis had taken a seat on the end of the pew. Dad sat in his wheelchair in the aisle, on Dennis's left. Mom sat on his right. They had saved a space for me.

I dragged a chair from the foyer, and settled in it, just inside the sanctuary door. The church seemed smaller than I remembered it. Everything seems smaller when you've been to the other side of the world and back, even the people. I recognized some of the congregation. They were healthy, vibrant adults in my memories. Now, like my parents, the women were getting shorter and a little humped, the men thicker around the middle and moving like their hip joints were frozen.

There were the same two rows of dark pews separated by a single aisle covered with carpet so old there was a bare spot running down the middle of it. The floor seemed to creak and sway a little with the weight of this joyous homecoming crowd.

The pulpit was not the massive hand-hewn piece of work I remembered. One of the founding members of Asbury Methodist, a man who lived in Oak Grove before the Civil War, had built it using handmade tools. When I was a kid, I used to sneak up there when the church was empty, rub my shirtsleeve on the varnished wood and try to see my reflection. It felt like a door to the past, like I had touched something that had touched someone's hands who had touched someone else's hands forming a chain that extended backward in time for as far back as generations could reach, maybe even to Adam and Eve.

I had forgotten how good heartfelt music could sound, singing that was untrained, unpracticed, with the women blending their soprano and alto with the men's tenor and baritone. There were no operatic high notes at Asbury Methodist, no melodramatic bass runs in this church. There were just good, solid people, staying between the lines, making pretty music, living lives of moderation, happy to be here.

I relaxed a little. I looked at Dennis, singing like he hadn't missed a Sunday in years. I started to hum along, careful not to make enough noise to draw any attention toward me.

From time to time, Dennis would turn and wave at me, or Mom would look back at me and frown, then look down at the empty space beside her, like she was trying to move me by the power of her will from my chair near the foyer into the pew with my family. I managed to avoid eye contact.

Finally, the preacher put his Bible on the lectern and read, "Let not your heart be troubled." I remembered that line. I didn't know where it was in the Bible, or what came before it or after it, but I knew those words by heart. When I told Dad I had orders for Vietnam, he wrote the whole verse down on the back of an envelope and tucked it in my shirt pocket. It always made me sad, so I quit reading it. It felt good to reach in my pocket and feel it though. I lost it, somewhere along the way.

As the preacher read, I noticed Dad kept twisting in his chair, trying to look back over one shoulder, then the other. Dennis kept rubbing his arm, and Mom leaned over and whispered to him. He ignored them, craned his head around, twisting, turning, staring over and through all those people he had known all his life as if he didn't know who they were or where he was. He had developed a tremor with his mental decline, and it got worse when he was flustered. His Bible flopped in his hands as if it was alive. He twisted himself even further in his chair. He looked straight at me, and stuttered, aloud, interrupting the preacher, "Don't... worry." I wasn't sure if he was summarizing the verse or trying to tell me that things were going to get better.

I ran down the aisle as he lurched to his feet. I reached him as his eyes glazed over. Dennis and I caught him as he started to fall.

The preacher stopped preaching and prayed, "God be with Ewell. Be with Tommy and Dennis and Della, too, in Jesus name, amen." Then he had the song leader start the congregation singing "When the Roll is Called Up Yonder," to keep them occupied, I guess.

Dad roused a little, studied me for a moment. He looked at Dennis, then at Mom. I couldn't tell if he was happy or sad, whether he knew us or not. He closed his eyes and looked like he went to sleep. I propped his feet on a stack of song books to let the blood flow to his brain. I folded his hands on his belly, farmer's hands with knobby knuckles, cracked fingernails, and big ropy veins. Dennis folded his sport coat under Dad's head, then leaned over him like he was looking for something in Dad's eyes, their profiles almost identical, mirror images.

Doc Haskins met us in the emergency room. "Good to see you boys again," he said as he hugged my mom. He shook my hand without flinching, then Dennis's without fawning. I could see Mom's anxiety disappear even before he listened to Dad's heart and lungs with his antique stethoscope.

"Ewell's had another stroke, Della," Doc said as he checked Dad's reflexes with a small rubber hammer.

Mom nodded. I had the feeling they had talked about this before. She may have told me.

"It'll be a merciful thing if he doesn't wake up." Doc looked at Mom. "We can keep him here in the hospital, but there is nothing I can do here that you can't do at home."

That line suggesting a merciful death surprised me. I've been so low I thought I'd be better off dead, too, and I didn't like the feeling. Dad didn't look like the prospect bothered him very much.

Mom's hands were fidgeting at her waist, feeling for her apron strings. At home, she kept them looped around her, tied in a bow on her belly. She moved a wisp of gray hair that escaped from the bun on the back her neck.

"We'll take him home, Doc." She looked like she might cry. She had that same look the Sunday I left for Fort Campbell, the day Dennis and I went our separate ways.

We stood on either side of Dad's bed, Dennis and me. I could hear Mom in the kitchen, clanking dishes, cooking and cleaning. That's what she did when she was happy. It's what she did when she was sad. "Everything and everybody I love comes to me through this kitchen," she said.

Dad had started to labor with his breathing over the evening. Doc had given him an injection of something in the emergency room, and I suspected it was starting to wear off. I heard him tell Mom he would come out tonight if we needed him. That made me feel better. Dad was breathing in a rhythm that was first loud, rapid and deep, then soft, slow and shallow, followed by several seconds of no breathing at all. After that, he'd start the cycle again.

I could tell the pauses scared Dennis. He still thought death was just what happened when the breathing stopped. He didn't know it takes effort to die. He didn't know the taste of a gun barrel on his tongue, the feel of metal on the back of his throat, the humiliation of not having the courage to finish.

"He'll start back," I said, even though each pause seemed to last a little longer. "It's his brain damage that makes him breath that way." I felt self-conscious, explaining this to my educated brother. "Doc Haskins told me," I added, even though he hadn't. I had seen it in the some of the old veterans at the VA domiciliary, and asked one of the interns what caused it.

"He doesn't know me," Dennis said.

"He's pretty bad off," I said. "I doubt if he knows anything right now."

"No. I mean he doesn't know me, doesn't know who I am."

Dennis sounded like me talking to myself late at night.

"He was proud of you," Dennis said. "He mailed me newspaper clippings every time there was a write-up about you." He reached down and rubbed his finger in an outline of an eagle tattooed on Dad's wasted upper arm, the unit crest for the 101st Airborne division. I had the same one on my shoulder.

"Pretty intimidating to have a brother who single-handedly made the world safe for democracy." He smiled a little, the smile he used to give when he had won some award, took first place in something, a smile that said he wasn't really sure if he had won it on his merits, or just won it like a lottery, by chance. He was always modest, always seemed a little guilty at his successes. I had forgotten.

Dennis continued, "He never was happy with me just going to law school. I think he was glad I went, but sometimes I think he wanted me to join up after I graduated, even though the war was over, just to pay my dues."

The only noise in the room was Dad's raspy breathing. His farmer fingers picked aimlessly at the edge of his blanket.

"He was proud of you," I said. "He showed me your office building once."

Dad coughed a weak, wet, rattling cough.

"Do you think he can hear us?" Dennis asked.

"Wouldn't surprise me," I said. We watched him cycle through his breathing again.

"Tell me about him showing you my office," Dennis said.

"We went to Knoxville for something, and he was driving around real slow downtown. I was just out of the hospital, so I thought he was trying to keep me occupied. I noticed he kept looking up at the buildings, especially the tallest ones. He was muttering, shaking his head. He finally parked the truck there on Gay Street and just sat looking up at one building in particular, not saying anything, like he was admiring the glass and chrome. We must have sat there a half hour before he started the truck and pulled out onto the street again. 'That's Dennis's building,' was all he said. He said it like you owned the place."

Dad was in the harsh cycle of his breathing, which was a blessing. It kept the silence at bay, kept some noise between Dennis and me so we could stand without needing to talk.

"I didn't know things were this bad," Dennis said as the breathing became softer and faded again. "I wish Mom had told me."

"You couldn't have changed anything, even if you'd known," I said. "She didn't tell me as much as you'd think." I was glad she hadn't. Sometimes not knowing is a good thing. Sometimes, no memory at all is better than a bad one.

"Does Mom still predict snowstorms?"

I told him there was a calendar hanging on the refrigerator with all the fogs during this August already marked. Several seconds of silence passed before Dad started breathing again.

"Do they still have that record player?" Dennis asked, keeping his eyes on Dad.

Mom kept a collection of albums, waltzes and marches, anything mass-produced in the sixties by a generic orchestra or band, anything sold at Sears. There was usually a scratch on the record that almost kept the beat whether the orchestra played "Tales of the Vienna Woods" or "The Stars and Stripes Forever."

I had watched them on clear nights, from my bedroom window. It was different from what I knew Dennis was remembering, when Dad swept Mom about the room with wild, homemade dance steps that left both of them breathless. The last time I watched, their shadows kind of held onto each other, and Mom was leading him around the room. Her steps were tiny, tentative, and Dad followed her in rhythm to some melody that I could feel all the way up to my cabin, but one only he and Mom could hear.

"They still danced, sometimes," I said, "until he got so feeble."

I looked out the window, up the hill, toward my cabin. The trees, shrubs, fences were just gray silhouettes, like an old black and white photograph. The clouds had made a halo around the moon. Downstairs, I could hear Mom singing "Where the Roses Never Fade." I leaned over Dad, felt his sour breath blow over me. I got closer and closer, till my face was almost touching his. I could almost see my reflection in his eyes.

The Diving Bell

Mona's blonde hair curled around her face in moist ringlets, still wet from her third shower of the day, still smelling sweet of Prell shampoo. She liked the fresh feeling, the clean smell of soap. She knew it wouldn't last long. Illness permeated her house, saturated the air making it so thick it was hard to breathe. She imagined that her clothes carried odors from dank, dark places, basement smells, and stagnant moisture. Everything she cooked tasted like it was spoiled, and made her gag. Already slender, she had lost twenty pounds in in the past six weeks. Her hands were chapped from washing. The pale area that marked the absence of her wedding band was almost invisible.

She stooped to examine the plastic bag that drained Bruce's bladder. The urine was dark, concentrated, and smelled like the rotten egg odor that used to nauseate her when she hurried by the chemistry lab at school. She lifted the catheter threaded into his penis. As the last drops of moisture drained into the bag, he groaned and wrinkled his forehead.

"I'm sorry, Honey Bunch," she said. She had insisted that everyone call him Bruce, but even she couldn't keep from using baby talk now. He looked so helpless, lying in a fetal position with drool puddling on a blue pad under his head. He hadn't talked to her in a week. Occasionally, when she was in another part of the house ironing or washing dishes, she would hear him mumble. There was never a sense of urgency in his voice, nothing that resembled her name. Still, when he made a sound, she went to him as faithful as an echo.

Mona fingered a small button that controlled the compact medicine pump lying by Bruce's pillow. The pump fed a catheter that carried morphine to a needle embedded under the loose skin of his belly. A tiny motor made a humming sound while it delivered the medicine Bruce needed to be comfortable. The nurses obsessed over the little machine, calculated how much extra Mona had given him, how much to adjust the background dose, like there was an equation to define the difference between comfort and discomfort, as if it were possible that he might upset some delicate balance and get too comfortable.

"Give it to him before he hurts," the hospice nurse said. "Don't let the pain build up until he's miserable. You'll use less medicine that way."

Mona had tiptoed reluctantly onto that slippery slope. It was hard, after his mind was gone, to act on her interpretation of his wrinkled forehead, his groans, his agitation. There were times that she imagined a missile hurtling toward Bruce's heart in response to her reluctant pressure on the control. The thought of it now made her press it again, as if to send a drop of morphine as reparation for the times when she hadn't given it only because she didn't know better.

Bruce had lost his vision before he lost his mind. He was still curious about the world, and insisted that Mona read him newspapers, magazines, books. Anything was fine, at first. It was odd how the scriptures seemed to give him peace after a while, odder still that she grew bitter and read without hearing anything more than words, empty of meaning. She was the one who grew up in the Oak Grove Baptist church, memorized the Ten Commandments, lived by the Golden Rule. He was the unchurched college professor with an intuitive sense of morality as pure

and unyielding as the Old Testament. Even now, her parents seemed unwilling to reconcile that his avoiding Vietnam had nothing to do with the injuries Mona's brother
suffered there. They rarely visited, usually stood in the living room and peered through the bedroom door at Bruce,
then left while reminding Mona that their whole church
was praying for them.

Still, she read to him as if she expected him to hear,
as if he might wake and want to discuss whatever the author was trying to say. Tonight, she read a story about a
scientist in the 1940s who studied the ocean floor by working in a diving bell. He described how he was constantly
afraid, how sometimes he wanted to scream through the
radio for the crew to drag him back to the surface because
he was running out of air. Mona looked outside at the oily
darkness, imagined the powerful sway of black water washing around them. Bruce just stared into the distance like he
was watching something in eternity.

Mona straightened her T-shirt and took in a long
breath, then dabbed a little Vaseline on Bruce's upper lip
where the friction of the plastic nosepiece had a blister going. His black hair budded in irregular patches all over his
head, the marks of chemotherapy and radiation finished
more than a month ago. His ratty beard emerged from
creases in the loose skin where his jawbones created an-
gles too sharp for her to give him a clean shave. He looked
much older than thirty-five, as old as one of those prehis-
toric men he described in his anthropology class, all forehead, eyebrows and jawbone.

The nurse had insisted on the oxygen, had placed a
long clear tube to puff it into Bruce's nostrils. "Don't worry," she assured Mona. "It won't prolong things. We only
do it to make him more comfortable."

"So the oxygen just fools his brain into believing
he's breathing?" Mona asked, her first open display of re-

sentment. "He doesn't know the difference, and he won't live longer?"

"Yes...I mean, I guess so." The nurse smiled as if this was a breakthrough, a terrific insight that she and Mona would use as a foundation to support a new relationship. "That's great, the way you sum things up, Mona. That must be from your training as a teacher." She smiled, encouraging Mona to continue the flow of feel-good banter.

"So why bother?" Mona asked. She regretted the word "bother" as it passed her lips. The nurses overanalyzed everything she said, found some deep emotional or psychological root to every word. When Mona was reluctant to give Bruce his pain medicines, it wasn't because she had a genuine fear of hurting him; it was because doing so would have her admit he was dying. She touched her wedding ring, now pinned to Bruce's pillow. They had interpreted that as an ominous signal and ignored the sore on her finger where her ring collected moisture.

The nurse rolled her mournful brown eyes. "Oh, Mona," she sighed. "We just want to improve his quality of life."

That's what she had hoped to do by moving to Oak Grove. She missed the sense of family, the mountains, the rivers, the small-town feeling of one grocery store, one post office, and no shopping mall. She wanted to force her parents to get to know Bruce the way she did, to understand that he was not a bad person.

They rented this small house on the edge of town, even though her job at the grade school was only part-time, even though living in Oak Grove created a long commute to the community college in Knox County where Bruce would teach. From the porch, she could see the steeple on the Baptist church she attended when she was young, the high school where she played basketball well enough to get a scholarship to the University of Virginia, the hosiery mill where both her parents worked, the entrance to the mines where both her grandfathers died before she was born. Bruce was unpacking his books when he had the seizure, went from healthy to unhealthy in that brief spasm, from a man brimming with life to someone who was slowly dying.

The specialists in Knoxville gave up a month ago, turned Bruce over to a bunch of do-good hospice nurses, an overweight chaplain, and to Doc Haskins, the same small-town GP who birthed Mona, patched her cuts and scrapes, gave her school vaccinations, did her college physical. Even back then, he talked so softly she could hardly hear him.

When Bruce started to choke on his own saliva, the doctor whispered that Bruce's brain couldn't coordinate his swallowing, that he would aspirate vomit into his lungs unless they placed a tube into his stomach so they could keep it suctioned dry. Now, the stomach tube emptied into a plastic container with milliliter markings on the side. Mona was supposed to give the nurses a record of how much fluid came out of Bruce every twenty-four hours, as if there was a data bank somewhere that pooled information from all over the country, forwarded it to a clearinghouse where some bureaucrat kept track of thick green yuck aspirated per person, per day, per year, per lifetime. Sometimes Mona made up numbers, large impossible volumes. No one ever questioned. It was just "palliative" care after all, not intended to make Bruce live longer, only to keep him comfortable.

The hospice chaplain had visited this evening. The meddling nurse had sent him over after the oxygen comment; Mona was sure of it. She probably called and pretended to be worried that poor Mona was experiencing a spiritual crisis, was wandering in her search for meaning.

He had surprised Mona during her evening shower. He stood on her porch with his black leather King James Version under his arm and knocked and knocked in the hot September dusk, long after an ordinary visitor would have taken the hint. She finally retreated into the washroom, dressed from the dirty clothes hamper, thinking he might leave if she came to the door with her hair wrapped in a towel.

"There is always hope," he had preached. His beatific eyes implied the thought was original, and he was overwhelmed at his own insight. He might just as well have said that the eye is like a camera for all the impact it had on Mona. "Hope is a changing, dynamic thing that evolves with an illness," he continued.

False hope to no hope, Mona thought.

"It was appropriate for you and Bruce to hope for a cure when you first learned of this tumor." He never said the word cancer. He claimed it called back painful memories of his wife's death. "It would be foolish to hope for that now," he said. He poked on Bruce's mattress with the square end of his index finger, as if it was a pulpit, as if he was preaching to a sanctuary full of interested listeners. "You should hope that however long we have Bruce, we can keep him comfortable."

The chaplain droned on while she wiped Bruce's lips with a washcloth, let him absorb some of the moisture. His breath smelled like rotting food, a sickening sweet odor like he was already dead on the inside.

"Or that Mona could find some measure of peace in her care giving role for Bruce," he continued.

Mona's caregiving role...the anger that had simmered in her for weeks started to boil. It would be a wonderful measure of peace if pious people would quit gushing profound phrases and offer to suction the snot out of his throat, to maybe clean the crap off his bottom, to help with all the unnatural things she had to do just because of that wedding ring pinned to his pillow.

When she tuned the chaplain in again, he was summarizing, shaping his sermon into a perfectly symmetric package, repeating the beginning at the end, neatly wrapping all the garbage in the middle. "We can always hope," he concluded.

Her emotional responses had become exaggerated, unpredictable. She had no control over how she might respond in any given situation, by crying or cursing, screaming or sulking.

"You don't know a thing about hope, you fat... you bastard ass," she said. Her voice trembled. She couldn't even swear fluently.

The chaplain sat with his fat hands folded in his lap like a nondenominational protestant Buddha figure carved in blubber.

"It's always good to let things out, Mona," he said. "It don't bother me none. I know it's Bruce's illness talking through you."

She looked at Bruce. This was not the man she married. This was not the athlete who ran, biked, and swam with her, not the teacher who made her think about things she had accepted as fact since childhood and let her question them without guilt. This was not that man. This skinny frame could easily be an artifact excavated from one of the Indian mounds in the mountains around Oak Grove. Nothing could talk through it.

"It's OK to be angry. It's even OK to be angry with your God." She noted his triumphant smile, knew he was revving up again. "He or She is big enough to let you be angry with Him or Her." He would launch into another sermon if she let him.

"I don't have a god," she said, hoping he would clutch his chest and fall to the floor where she would watch him writhe and clutch at her ankles while she leisurely dialed 911. "He, she, or it."

Her chest felt tight. She had to breathe in short, shallow puffs. The chaplain smiled and tried to pat her hand across the bed, then stood and bent over Bruce to say something sanctimonious. Mona stuck out her tongue at his enormous butt, caught a glimpse of her contorted face in the mirror on the dressing table. She ran to the bathroom rather than have the chaplain think he said something that had moved her to tears. Mona stepped into the shower without undressing, turned the hot stinging pellets of water full in her face. She stood there until her heart started to slow its angry rhythm, until she was certain the chaplain was gone, until she sensed that Bruce was calling out for her again.

He looked comfortable. He almost looked serene, the way he looked early in the mornings before he was sick, when the weight of her gaze would rouse him as she studied his sleeping profile. She turned the bed lamp off. Darkness swirled around them. She pulled back the sheet, and with her free hand still clutching the morphine button, curled her body next to his. From time to time, she rested her head on his chest and listened for an echo from the bottom.

ASHES TO ASHES

The smell of fresh coffee wending up the stairs and under my bedroom door surprised me. I thought my family had retired earlier in the evening, leaving me to study alone in my room. The smell intensified, coaxing me into the hallway. I tiptoed down the corridor where my mom's voice stopped me just at the creaky part of the stairs.

She sounded animated, even happy. I peeked around the corner. She was sitting with her chair pulled close to the kitchen table where she had centered two urns that I knew contained the ashes of her parents. She leaned toward them, elbows planted on either side of her coffee cup, chin resting on her folded hands, concentrating. She seemed at ease, without the worry lines that had wrinkled the corners of her eyes for the past months.

I didn't know that she ever moved the urns from the mantle until I saw her in conference with them in the kitchen. Wesley, my brother, had whispered to me that they contained "dead people ashes" years before. He assured me that the urns could move about the house under supernatural power. I think he sometimes moved them slightly, making sure that I noticed it later. Wide-eyed and fearful, he professed ignorance, cataloguing the incident as more evidence of their mystical abilities. Actually, the thought of those urns levitating through the house terrified me, even as a junior in high school. Some nights, I could feel them hovering over me in the dark.

I continued to eavesdrop. Mom and the urns, or rather the spirits in them, appeared to be talking about my father. I knew she had taken him to the doctor. He had lost weight so fast that he had cinched his belt up one notch every other week after Christmas. When it looped nearly halfway around him, he agreed to go.

"The Doctor made him swallow some of that dye so he could take pictures of his sarcophagus." Mom studied the urns like she expected them to answer her. Then she actually chuckled. It irked me that she seemed so happy when I hadn't heard her laugh in months. "OK. Esophagus... his swallowing tube. You know how I am with words. Doc Haskins says there's barely a trickle getting through there."

We had watched him eat more slowly, chew his food more thoroughly, and drink vast amounts of water to wash it down. His ritual had grown so labored and painful that he quit coming to the kitchen. We would listen to him in the living room, coughing, gagging, and struggling to get enough calories to sustain him one more day at the hosiery mill. Wesley would sit, fork in hand, unable to eat. Mother would fix a cold washcloth at the sink, then join my dad.

"Yes. We did talk about surgery. Doc says it won't help. He said we could send him to Knoxville to get some cobalt treatments, but the side effects might kill him faster than the cancer. I told him Roscoe had started drinking again. Doc said not to fuss with him. Said he might've started it to help ease the pain. He told me that when he gets down and can't swallow, to let him know and he would either make house calls or show me how to give him a hypodermic injection. I don't know why he can't give him morphine now. I reckon Doc is trying to save it for the end when he really needs it."

A long silence intervened, with my mother swaying slightly, listening attentively, and nodding her head occasionally. Suddenly, she stiffened, as if the conversation had veered in another direction. She pointed at one of the urns.

"Look, Mom, I'm sorry. I can't make Mrs. Miller do anything about that old tree. It's the same excuse. Her granddaddy stuck a walking stick in the ground a hundred years ago, and it took root. She can't bear to cut it down. She don't care that it's leaning over our porch. It's going to fall with the next big storm. She told me I can have the limbs trimmed back, long as I don't kill it, but that's all."

Mom kept talking to the urns long after I retreated to my bedroom, vaguely uneasy at how normal this seemed. I sat for hours by my window in the dark, watching the moon move in a slow arc across the sky before I heard her tiptoe down the hall to the bed she shared with my dad.

She didn't tell Wesley or me that Dad had cancer. I started sitting with them in the evenings anyway, after he became too weak to get out of bed. My mom kept him comfortable with whiskey, dosing him as precisely as an anesthesiologist until he became too weak to swallow. She spoke to me as an equal, a fellow conspirator, as if she was conveying information not suitable for the public.

"Physical pain ain't the problem," she said, spooning liquor onto my father's lips. "Physical pain and suffering ain't the same thing. It's possible to suffer and not feel the first twinge of physical pain. The body has a way of dealing with that. Remember ole man Cox cut off his left hand with a chain saw and managed to bandage it and drive to Knoxville to the hospital by himself. Didn't feel no pain till they started sticking needles in him to numb him up. Physical pain is what you talk about, what you try to relieve. Suffering's what's left when you get rid of the pain. It's what makes you walk the floor at night."

Mom moved the urns from the downstairs mantle to the dresser next to her bed. She no longer tried to hide her conversations with her parents. She would tell me things her mother had said, and even ask me if I could hear her talking.

"Mom," I thought, as I smiled at the shorter urn and pretended to listen. "I can't hear your hallucinations."

Mom's inability to separate her dead family from her living one frightened me. Her lengthy speeches about pain and suffering smothered me. When our big old creaky house seemed smaller, I started sleeping with my window open. The wind fluttering the curtains and ruffling my bedclothes kept me from suffocating.

By May, the wintergreen smell of liniment and whiskey burned my lungs with every breath I took. Doctor Haskins started making his house calls. As if by some supernatural signal, when Dad would start to moan, Doc would slip in the front door. The stairs creaked under his weight. His black bag clinked with vials, syringes and needles. Mom called it the art of medicine, the transcendent communication of one who suffers to one who relieves it. Sometimes, Doc would sit with Mom for a while as the morphine took effect. Then he would leave, with not a single word passing between them.

On his final visit, Doc must have wondered how long after my dad died that Mom had sat there talking with him. He couldn't have known that she had become so other-worldly that she didn't notice little things, like the exit of life from the body. He didn't even try to close my dad's eyelids, frozen open, his gaze fixed on a focal point an eternity away. Doc took one of Mom's hands in both of his, mumbled his condolences, picked up his black bag and left.

Wesley graduated from high school that spring. Two days after Dad died, one week before Mom placed the third urn on the dresser, he packed his bag and joined the Army. He and Mom held hands, said goodbye, and promised to write. He turned to me, kissed the top of my head and walked out the door. I never saw him again.

Mom changed even more after Wesley left. She rarely smiled, but she always looked serene. She talked over me, in another realm. A simple question would prompt a rambling answer. A statement would provoke an ethereal question of premise.

From the street, we still appeared to be normal. Our yard looked beautiful save for the oak tree teetering over the edge of the house. Flowers of all hues grew along our sidewalk, implying a levity that didn't exist. The people of Oak Grove admired our ability to cope.

The window to our adjacent bedrooms overlooked the gently sloping roof that covered the front porch. At night before Dad died, I would crawl out there. I had to step over the tree limbs that so frustrated my mother. That was the only place that I could escape the stale odor of liniment and the weighty speeches about suffering. After Dad died, I kept doing it. The heat stored in those shingles seeped through my clothes, deep into the muscles of my back and rejuvenated me. Down the roof, I could see the faint glimmer of light from my mom's bedroom. I pictured her rocking, talking and listening to the spirits in the three urns. Then, I would look up and try to count the stars and feel so insignificant and humble that I imagined I could feel a mass growing in my own chest that only crying relieved.

One morning, in the spring of 1969, Mom came down to the kitchen where I sat eating cereal and said, "Wes came home last night."

I knew better. He'd left Fort Campbell two months before. We both had letters from Vietnam describing his arrival there. He had tried to make it sound like a field trip.

"He was here," she insisted. "He stood at the end of my bed and shook it till I woke up. He had on his dress uniform. He had his jump boots shined so bright that the reflection of the moon lit up the whole room. He was so close I could see the eagle's head patch on his left shoulder. He kept looking, and looking, then he saluted, then his body faded, from the feet up. Last thing I saw was his eyes."

Later, I heard her talking to the urns. "Did you see him? He stood right here, in this room. You had to see him."

Silence.

"Do you know if he's alive?"

Silence for a long while.

"I'm tempted to flush you all down the toilet for the good you are. I should've buried you like the mortician told me."

Mom spent her days waiting for the mailman after that. She seemed to move in a fog. Any movement required great effort. Minimal exertion caused tiredness so profound she'd go to bed in the afternoon and not get up for hours. The smell of food cooking made her nauseous. Weeds took over her flowerbeds. Garbage piled up in the wastebaskets. A layer of dust coated the furniture. My attempts to help only made her sink to the nearest chair and cry.

After a month and no letters from Wesley, Mom took to her bed for good. She just lay there, facing her three urns, each day turning a little more transparent than the day before. She wouldn't let me call Doc Haskins.

I left toast and coffee for her in the mornings as I left for school. When I returned, they had grown cold, untouched, on her bedside table. I sat with her, but she rarely acknowledged my presence. She took no medicine, but my imagination conjured up the smell of liniment and whiskey again. I didn't like that smell or the feeling.

Mom grew heavier as she faded, needing more and more assistance in moving from the bed to bathroom, then bed to chair, then from side to side. The night she died, her body sagged further into the bed linens than it ever did in life. Before she stopped breathing, her face had frozen into a mask, her lips into a thin hard line, as if she had to solve a complicated math equation. Her translucent white skin stretched tight over high cheekbones and sunk deeply inward at the temples. She looked like a statue in repose, a relief carved in ivory. I reached to feel for her pulse, but my hand changed direction in midair. Instead, I adjusted her wedding band so that the tiny diamond faced outward.

I sat by her bed, looking from her toward the three urns, imagining that the spirits inside them could see me. I wondered if my brother, lost on patrol in the spirit world, knew she had died, maybe even before I found her. I felt like an intruder.

The wind stirred the curtains at her bedroom window, fluttered at me in a distinctly beckoning manner. I stepped over and opened the window wide. The smell of new rain entered. I took several deep breaths of the cool, clean air. The limbs of the old oak tree scraped on the roof. The bulk of the tree was visible only as an outline in the darkness.

The wind gusted again. One side of the curtain literally circled my hand, as if to lead me through the open window. I kicked off my loafers, hiked up my skirt and climbed out onto the roof. I moved down, away from the window. The shingles bit into my bare feet. I resisted the urge to look back at Mom and stretched out on my back. Heavy clouds raced across the sky, making the night alternate in pitch black darkness and hazy gray fog. A few raindrops sprinkled over me before the wind blasted a salvo of water against the far side of the house. The clouds continued to fly overhead, dropping their munitions on me in waves.

Lightning bolts played across the sky in short zapping darts of light, spending their energy high in the air.

Thunder clapped somewhere above Knoxville and traveled south over me, grumbling all the way to Chattanooga.

Then, just as suddenly as it started, the rain stopped. The clouds cleared and a few stars twinkled among the clouds. I started to experience the spinning, vertiginous sensation of falling upward, into the sky. I may have slept, but not for long.

The evening peace exploded with a long, jagged bolt of lightning that scorched the roof on the far end of the house filling the air with a smell of burned tar. The shadow in the dark that had once been the majestic oak tree disappeared.

I stood carefully, trying to steady myself at the windowsill and wring water from my skirt. I straightened, straining in the dark to detect storm damage to the far corner of the house. Finally, satisfied that the tree had been demolished without ruining the porch, I prepared to step back through the window. The glow from Mom's bed lamp reflected off the three brass urns, illuminating her face. I had forgotten how she looked when she smiled.

This Old House

An evening breeze rustled the trees, stirring leaves destined to die. Claire snuggled a patchwork quilt tight over her legs and hunched her bony shoulders against the chill of the autumn evening. Greg leaned on the porch rail with his arms folded, his legs crossed at the ankles like a teenage catalog model. The thin spot in the middle of his too-long, gray hair was hidden by a baseball cap pushed back on his head. Claire turned her gaze to the faded red, T-top Corvette in the gravel drive.

"Why did you do this?" She picked at the frayed edge of her coverlet.

"Why not?" he answered.

"Where did you get the money?"

"The bank," he said. "They have a tree. I picked a handful."

"That's not funny," Claire said, surprised at the strength of her own voice. She thought of the medical bills piled on the kitchen table.

"It's a '69," Greg said.

"So?" she asked. "The porch is about to fall off the front of the house. The yard looks like the Air Force uses it for bombing practice." The hard edge in her voice faded with each word. "We have bills to pay," she whispered. "What were you thinking?"

She had read in a magazine about women with distorted body images, skinny women who starved themselves because, when they looked in the mirror, they thought themselves fat. *Greg must have a distorted life image*, she thought, *one that doesn't let him see reality.* He looked in the mirror and thought he had money. He looked at Claire and didn't see that she was dying.

"It's the year we won State," he said. A smile flickered across his face at the memory.

"It's the year we were married," Claire said.

Greg didn't acknowledge her. "And this old house ain't worth what it would cost to fix, anyway," he said.

That's not what you said when we bought it, she thought. It was a real fixer-upper back then.

Greg stared at her as if to say, "Your move."

"We don't have money to make payments on a worn-out car," Claire said.

"It's not worn out. It's a classic."

Greg hesitated, as if he wanted to say something more. Instead, he walked past Claire, across the porch, and down the swaybacked, creaking steps.

"I've gotta get to the field," he said.

Greg had volunteered years ago to maintain the scoreboard and stadium lights for the high school football team. He said it kept him near the game. The starter whined before the engine caught. Greg revved the motor as he backed into the street. An oil spot on the gravel marked the place where he had parked.

Claire stood, stretched, leaned on the porch railing, and felt it sag a little. Greg was lucky it hadn't collapsed and dumped him into the yard. A warning tingle started behind her ears. She adjusted her lilac-colored chemo turban. A hint of breeze on her scalp would cause it to erupt into a tingling itch begging her to scratch.

She went into the living room, settled into her Barclay recliner, and washed down two Percocet with a mouth full of stale coffee. *When did I leave it here? This morning? Last night?* She looked around. There were cups all over the room, either empty or with a nauseating skim over the top of whatever liquid remained. Time had become a matter of perspective. Ten a.m. only meant it was two hours until her next scheduled pain pill. December was almost three refills away.

Her stomach churned. She closed her eyes and waited for the feeling to pass. She took an extra pill and without thinking, lifted the cold coffee to her lips again. She gagged, swallowed, and gagged again.

"Just take it when you hurt," Doc Haskins had said. "It unhooks your mind from your body, so you don't perceive pain as something bad."

She checked her bottle. The medicine was so powerful that the law only let him write for one month at a time. Claire was terrified at the thought of running out. She had heard horror stories at the clinic about people who lost their bottles or misjudged when they would need more or somehow created the impression that they were irresponsible, causing their doctor to refuse to authorize a refill. She had accumulated a small stockpile by overreporting her pain, and after one of her fellow patients died, the family gave Claire a shoe box full of narcotic patches, tablets, and elixirs.

She settled back in the recliner, her thoughts fuzzy at the edges. The stadium lights at the high school glowed in the sky over Oak Grove. The silhouette of Roan Mountain squatted like a cat behind it. The crowd roared from time to time, usually followed by the frantic metallic rhythms of the Oak Grove Miners marching band. She took another pill and tried to unhook herself from the cancer that had latched onto her for life.

Greg had cried when Doc Haskins told them that the tiny melanoma he removed from Clair's shoulder three years earlier had recurred.

"It's in your liver," he said. "That's why you hurt under your rib cage."

"But...I thought they got it all," Claire said. Doc had sent her to a surgeon, who took a huge divot around the place where he had excised the original tumor. She fingered the scar through her blouse.

"There's a small percentage of people whose tumor comes back, anyway," he said. Doc's rheumy, old eyes looked sadder than usual. "I'll send you to a specialist in Knoxville," he said. "Maybe he can buy us some time."

She felt Greg crying more than heard him, noticed in her peripheral vision that his shoulders where shaking and he was digging at his eyes with his knuckles, not just a moist-eyed token of manly concern but a humiliating demonstration of hopelessness and despair.

Yesterday, less than three months after the news from Doc Haskins, her oncologist hung her scans on a view box and pointed out the nodules scattered through her liver. They were easy to see.

"Some of these are larger. None of them are smaller," he said.

Claire didn't speak.

"The chemotherapy isn't working," he continued.

She still didn't speak.

He studied her as if trying to decide whether her silence meant she hadn't understood him or that she was too stunned to answer.

"I don't have any rabbits to pull out of my hat," he said. "I can send you somewhere for a clinical trial. I'm not enthusiastic, though. It's like donating your body to science before you die."

Claire wondered if Greg would cry when he heard this news.

The doctor continued, filling the air with words that crowded out her questions. "You need to be as comfortable and functional as you can be for whatever time you have," he said. The word "hospice" swirled to the surface of his monologue but quickly submerged again under the weight of his words.

"Hospice?"

"It's an operational definition," he said. "The law says if you only have a reasonable expectation of living six months or less, you qualify."

"Six months?" she asked, even though she knew. Her mind started to jumble the information. *There's a law?*

How can this be? She was still driving herself to his office. Sure…when the nausea meds were too sedating, the nurses made her sleep an extra hour, but she drove herself to and from every appointment. *Rabbits? Does he consider chemotherapy a magic trick? A clinical trial is worse than hospice?* Everything seemed backward.

The doctor was standing. "Any questions?" he asked. He smiled as if it caused his jaw to hurt.

"No," she said.

Claire walked out through the chemotherapy suite. A dozen people with a variety of cancers in an assortment of stages looked at her, then looked away. She had watched familiar faces come and go, then reappear in long obituaries with pictures and stories that didn't match what she thought she knew. The wormy little guy who cried every time the nurses put his needle in had been a prisoner of war in Japan in WWII. The lady who wore a Dolly Parton wig to cover her hair loss had retired after working thirty years behind the cosmetic counter at Rich's department store, a Miss Tennessee finalist in 1963.

Claire wondered what Greg would write in her obituary. All she had done was graduate from Oak Grove High School, marry Greg, earn a certificate from the Tennessee School of Beauty and cultivate varicose veins from standing in a hair salon day after day. She looked around the room, then left without saying goodbye.

Even now she wasn't sure what made her think breaking the news to Greg was best done at the store. She had started there straight from the doctor's office, then changed her mind. She went home and waited until almost closing time to drive down to see him. She sat in her car and watched through the store windows as an old man paid for his groceries, then wheeled them across the parking lot in a rickety wire shopping cart.

Greg came to the checkout lane with a clipboard in his hand. Claire noted the easy way the redheaded cashier leaned on his arm, how his hand lingered on her back when he moved behind her to cash out her register.

Claire looked away. Her eyes followed the ridge-line, where the warning light for low-flying aircraft blinked at the top of the fire tower. She and Greg had parked under that tower in high school and made promises to each other.

The moon hovered where the sun used to be, cold and gray as a burned-out charcoal briquette. Claire reconciled herself to the reality of recent months, even before she was sick, when she had wakened in the gray-fringed dawn with Greg's side of the bed cool to her touch.

She drove home and stretched out on her recliner. When Greg came in, she pretended to sleep.

She saw Doc Haskins the next day, who confirmed what the oncologist said. She spent the rest of the day with her mother at Shannondale on the Alzheimer's ward.

"Doc Haskins says I only have a month or two at the most," she said.

"Bless your heart," her mother answered while turning her face away from the spoonful of baby food Claire touched to her lips. She put the spoon on the tray and watched her mother fold and unfold a paper napkin.

"It's Alzheimer's more than depression," Doc said when the relentless decline after her father's death stretched from months to years. "She probably had the early stages while she was taking care of your dad, and we just couldn't see it."

Claire still wondered if the trauma of that death had triggered something in her mother's brain that turned the reality switch to "off."

"Mom..." she said. "Doc says he won't let me hurt. He'll make sure I have pain medicine."

She looked at Claire with the tantalizing glimmer of recognition in her eyes that faded as fast as it appeared. She smiled and folded the napkin again. "Bless your heart," she said.

The aroma of strong coffee woke Claire. The air was cold through the open window. Her blanket had slipped to the floor. She felt stiff, like someone had dipped her in paraffin while she slept. The lights were still on at the stadium, glowing in the sky like an alien's spaceship. The field house crew had to clean up after the game before Greg could turn everything off. Once, after the Miners had sealed the regional championship, he left the lights on all night, prompting the editor of the *Oak Grove Herald* to write a commentary exhorting the school board to be better stewards of the taxpayers' money. The board, in turn, told Greg there were other aging high school quarterbacks lined up, waiting for the opportunity to take his job.

She sat on the edge of the chair until the world leveled out, then gathered her ragged, pink, terry cloth bathrobe off the couch and draped it over her shoulders. She skimmed her fingers along the wall to steady herself while she walked into the kitchen.

Greg sat at the table, looking out the window. A swirl of steam curled off the edge of his cup. He was frowning.

Claire moved to the side window without speaking. A gray full moon made the night look colder. The Corvette's smooth, classic lines made a seductive shadow in the driveway.

She watched Greg's reflection in the window glass. He continued to stare into space, sipping his coffee and frowning. After he had drained the cup, he rubbed his eyes and combed his fingers through his hair.

"Let's go for a ride," he said.

He started toward the door, looked over his shoulder, made a subtle change in his gait that reminded Claire of Friday nights thirty years earlier, when his elusive moves made it nearly impossible for his opponents to hold him. "Come on," he said.

She didn't move.

He came back to her and took her arm. "I have to go back and shut down the lights."

They stopped in the living room while she stepped into her loafers. The movement made her hip hurt. She stood on one foot like a pelican. When the pain abated, she limped across the room. They walked across the creaky porch, down the rickety stairs, and down the path across the yard to the gravel drive. She leaned in the window, while Greg waited behind her. The leather seats were worn, and there were tears at the seams. A worn, fancy key ring with the Corvette imprint on it dangled from the ignition.

How could he borrow money for a worn-out car somebody had discarded to make room for their next midlife crisis? she wondered. *What was he thinking?*

Greg opened the door and stood aside. He held her arm while she settled carefully into the bucket seat, then he walked around the car and slipped under the steering wheel. The starter caught quickly. The motor settled into a grumbling idle.

He said something, but she couldn't hear him.

"What?" she said. Her voice cracked from trying to speak over the noise of the engine.

He reached across and snapped the seat belt across her lap. He backed into the street, and headed down Kingston Avenue, past the old Oak Grove aristocrats' homes. He stopped at the red light before crossing the boulevard that paralleled the railroad tracks and separated Oak Grove into halves.

They both looked down the street toward Archie's drive-in. It was still busy, even at this time of night. There were cars parked at the curb for service, and a steady line of old Chevrolets, Fords, Impalas, and Mustangs—all painted in loud colors, their bodies jacked up to accommodate tires that stuck out from under the rear fender wells, their engines loping at barely more than an idle—circling the place time and again.

The light changed. Greg hesitated, like he wanted to join the procession. Instead, he headed across the street and over the tracks. The car bumped, transmitting every jolt to Claire's sore bones. *This thing rides like a go-cart*, she thought. She wished she had a hand full of Percocet.

They drove through the residential area that surrounded the schoolgrounds, rows of old, small, white frame homes built when the coal company provided houses for its employees. The lights were bright, and televisions muted by closed windows played in every living room. They passed a grassy park with benches and a merry-go-round that had been just a patch of woods when she was young.

Greg turned onto the road that passed behind the stadium where the players entered, where the fire department parked the paramedic van during each game. The gate to the field was still open. She could see an old man mopping in the field house and a boy pushing a big canvas cart full of muddy towels.

Claire expected Greg to park the car and talk to the workers, then shut down the stadium lights and head home. Instead, he turned the car toward the field. The front of the corvette bucked across the running track. The rear fish-tailed in the grass as the wide bald tires searched for traction. Claire's stomach rolled. Greg finally stopped on the fifty-yard line with the front of the car pointed toward the home side of the stadium.

The world seemed quieter, brighter than it should, almost the way it felt three decades ago, when she stood on this same spot and accepted her crown as the Class of 1969, Oak Grove Miners homecoming queen.

Greg turned off the engine. He propped his right wrist on top of the steering wheel, his left elbow in the window. "I think I should move out," he said without any sort of preamble.

Claire didn't register what he said and looked across the field at the empty stands. She remembered the uniformed band members, elegant in stiff, wool suits with the too-tall hats and a feather on top that flipped and jerked one way or another, depending on the choreography. She pictured the cheerleaders high-kicking, jumping, tossing each other in the air, then talking earnestly among themselves between routines.

"I think I should move out," Greg said again.

She imagined the student section surrounded by the oblivious adults, all of them filling the air with disposable words, caught up in the contrived importance of a game between adolescent males from neighboring counties.

Greg was looking at her as if he had been talking for a while. "I need some time to myself," he said.

She looked up at the press box, heard the announcer chant like he did when Greg returned a punt. "He's at the twenty, he breaks a tackle at the thirty, he's across the forty-yard line, he's at the fifty and running free…"

"Time to yourself?" she asked.

"Time to himself," she answered.

"I'm just talking about staying somewhere else for a while," he said. "Just send the bills to the store. I'll take care of things from there."

"You'll be sleeping in the store?" Claire asked. She couldn't resist. She used to surprise him, show up at closing time wearing a skimpy, cotton sundress and nothing else, take his hand, lead him down the aisle, where they were barely out of sight of the storefront windows, and let her clothes fall away while she took off his. Afterward, they'd lie on the couch in his office and watch television on a 13-inch black-and-white screen until the sun came up.

The sun always came up back then.

"Yeah. I mean, sometimes. I guess not all the time, but that's where I am most of the time. I didn't think you'd want to talk to me at night."

Claire's face warmed. How could he not know that he was as transparent as a windshield? Oak Grove people didn't retreat to their lake house or their mountain cabin to sort things out. Oak Grove people just packed a change of clean underwear in a brown paper bag and transferred their stale hopes into somebody else's dream.

"During the day…it's the best place to get in touch with me is all I meant," he said.

The announcer's reference to Greg's running free echoed in her ears.

"I'm cold," she said.

Greg turned the ignition. The engine grumbled. He turned the heater on. The noisy fan blew hot air on her feet.

It seemed pointless to ask for more.

Span of Life

Doc Haskins fingered the frayed edges of the clinic file, remembering the details of BJ Isham's birth far more graphically than he could have ever recorded them. He rubbed his hand across his bald head, removed his wire rim glasses, and pinched the bridge of his nose. It would have been a difficult delivery even in a hospital, and should have been done by an obstetrician with surgical equipment and an assistant or two, even in 1965.

She was naked when he found her flat on her back, hands squeezing the edges of a filthy mattress, legs flailing, eyes brimming with fear, her mouth fixed to deliver a feral wail. While Doc was absorbing this picture, while he wondered how things could possibly be worse, he watched a little foot emerge from Jan's female parts, like a tiny person was testing the water temperature with its toe.

A few months before, Burl Isham had stood in the clinic, slack-jawed, unshaven, wearing filthy bib overalls. Jan stood a little to the side and behind Burl, her mouth stained with tobacco juice, her eyes casting anywhere she could look without having to meet someone's gaze.

Burl hadn't bothered to call for an appointment. He never did. He just appeared unannounced, always claimed that he and Doc had known each other too long for him to have to schedule a visit. Doc Haskins, son of the company doctor at the now-defunct Oak Grove Coal Works, had attended the first few years of school with Burl Isham, son of the town drunk. When Doc was 16, he went to college. When Burl was sixteen, he moved in with Jan, a thirty-year-old woman with the mind of a child.

Burl told the receptionist that Doc Haskins needed to run some tests on Jan to see if she was "that way." She'd lost a dozen other pregnancies, each diagnosed in a similar impromptu clinic visit. Jan never demonstrated behavior that indicated a maternal instinct and ignored his advice about prenatal care. They just disappeared with their diagnosis, only to reappear when she was pregnant again. In a town where mothers named their miscarried babies and had funerals for them, Doc imagined that Jan dropped hers in the outhouse with no more thought about it than a cat. He quit worrying about them eventually, assuming that God would not allow people so ignorant to complete a pregnancy.

Seven months later, Burl had skidded his dilapidated truck into the clinic parking lot, pounded up the front steps, waded through a full waiting room, and yelled to the receptionist, "Doc needs to git on out to the house, Jan's birthin' herself a baby." As much as Burl and Jan disgusted him, Doc had left an office full of people and drove into the country to deliver their baby.

Burl was waiting on him, windmilling one arm and then the other as if he could winch Doc into the yard. He was worthless after that, wouldn't lead him to Jan, wouldn't come into the house. Doc fought through the stench, followed the sound of her moaning to a bedroom with a bare mattress on the floor. He hoped for a millisecond that the baby would be stillborn, then feared simultaneously that Jan would break its neck with her thrashing. It was a cruel miracle that neither had happened already. Outside, Burl blustered up and down, his head appearing in the bedroom window every few minutes, his foul breath fogging the glass where he mouthed inane comments and questions about Jan's progress.

Doc managed to deliver the baby feet-first, cut the cord, and drop the placenta into a yellow plastic lard bucket that Burl used to pee in at night rather than walk to the outhouse. Then, with the infant snuggled in a blanket against his chest, proud of himself, proud of his profession, Doc turned to show him to Jan. She turned her face to the wall and gave no sign that she wanted to hold it, showed no interest in whether it was a boy or a girl.

Doc walked to the door where Burl squatted on his heels smoking. "It's a boy," he said. It seemed like somebody should know.

Burl sucked on his cigarette. "I figgered so," he said, "judging from the way she was carrying it."

Doc felt his cheeks start to warm. He figured so, indeed.

"Burl, drive over to the Crabtree's. Ask them to call an ambulance to come out, right away."

"How come? I ain't no doctor, but she looks OK to me. Why you gonna send 'er to the hospital?"

Doc glared at him. "Send *them*, Burl, your wife and your baby boy."

Burl skulked out to his truck and disappeared slowly down the drive. While he waited for the ambulance, Doc moved the baby to the kitchen table where he cleaned him with rags he found under the sink. He examined the tiny feet and hands, counted the fingers and toes, and listened to the little heart race. He worried about a good-sized bruise on the side of the boy's head, hoped it didn't signal worse news on the inside. As Doc worked, the baby rolled his eyes, yawned, and twisted his mouth into what almost looked like a crooked, whimsical grin, as if he wanted Doc to forgive his parents for their ignorance.

That newborn reflex was the only happy memory Doc had of BJ. He had tried to have the baby removed from the home, even offered to adopt him. Mrs. Haskins was agreeable, if not enthusiastic. They had no children of their own.

"I just worry," she said. "Burl's father was such a mean man." Her voice trailed away.

"I doubt if meanness is inherited," Doc said without conviction.

"And we both know how Jan came to be," she said.

Doc didn't answer. He had treated some of Jan's relatives, and he had strong clinical suspicions regarding incest in Jan's pedigree.

They were both relieved when the court declined their offer and didn't even question the bizarre notion that keeping BJ's "family unit" intact was best for him.

By the time BJ should have been in the eighth grade, Doc saw him regularly, as early as dawn, as late as midnight, walking aimlessly and alone, with his weak left arm flexed up tight, his left leg dragging, his head down, his skinny shoulders hunched, and his body hitching with every step. Sometimes, when he was making a house call, Doc would give him a ride, then drive out of his way to drop him at Burl's shack. BJ would exit the car and walk right by the house and head down the road to nowhere, as if anywhere was better than being at home.

Burl had stormed the clinic again today, twenty-five years older, but still wearing filthy overalls, muddy boots, still with facial hair that was something less than a beard but more than unshaven. He had told the receptionist, "Doc needs to come over. BJ's perty sick. He just got out of the hospital in Chattanooga."

"I can't get out there until my clinic is finished," Doc told him. "I can't just drop and run like I used to."

"I reckon that'll have to do," said Burl. "And us going back as far as we do."

While Doc struggled with the sense that he was needed in two places at once, his office nurse managed to have BJ's medical records faxed from the City Hospital in

Chattanooga. It was a far thicker file than a young man should have. There was a complicated hospital summary describing a month-long admission for treatment of pneumonia. Some of the notes listed BJ's medicines, new ones, with names Doc had never written on a prescription pad. Other entries documented his noncompliance, his failure to keep appointments, his inability to remember to take his medicines. The memory of BJ's aimless walking returned.

The sun was long gone when the last person left the clinic. Doc gathered the faxed records and picked up his black bag. It tinkled with empty glass medicine vials and syringes, more of a symbol than a necessity. The only important thing in it now was an index card with the phone numbers of the pharmacy, the ambulance service, and the only mortician in Oak Grove.

Doc enjoyed making house calls at night. As he wound his car down a country road, headlamps slicing through the darkness toward a farmhouse with a yellow light glowing on the front porch, stars twinkling, moon shining, the sensation was almost spiritual. He had never billed for a home visit, even when he was young. The cakes and pies, the gallons of hot coffee, and the adoration of grateful patients was enough. He always felt better even if the sick person didn't. Now, most of his home visits were with older folks, people who couldn't travel to town anymore, people he had treated for one thing or another for a half-century. He would sit with his empty medical bag on the floor next to his chair, a halo of white hair surrounding his head, his craggy face as furrowed as the worn-out farmland surrounding Oak Grove.

The drive from the clinic to Burl's house took less than half an hour. The January sky was cloudless, dark navy blue with white polka dot stars, and highlighted with a full moon, pure and white as a pearl pendant. He parked his jeep in the dirt near the front of Burl's place. A naked light bulb strained to illuminate the front porch. He stepped out and retrieved his bag from the front seat. A light flickered on in a window to one side of the front porch. Burl opened the door. Doc felt like he had stepped off the edge of a precipice.

"Evening Doc," Burl said. "Reckon you're tired. Been on the golf course all day, I bet."

Doc sighed. There wasn't a golf course in Oak Grove.

"The clinic was real busy today, Burl. I can't just leave it like I used to. Where's BJ?"

"He's sleeping," Burl said. "We woke up this morning an' there he was, in his bed, shivering like he was 'bout to die. Snuck in sometime during the night, I reckon. He ain't been home in months."

Doc didn't answer.

"I didn't know it was going to be so late when you got here. I almost called that new doctor over in Kingston Springs. But you and me go back so far, I just hated to."

Doc Haskins felt the skin on his neck get warm. There was no new doctor in Kingston Springs, either. He took a deep breath. "Take me to BJ," he said.

Burl coughed and wiped his nose on his sleeve. "I spread him a pallet in the front room close to the heater. He can't get warm."

Doc followed Burl through the door into a room where Jan sat by the window chewing on a cud of tobacco. An oil-burning stove stood in the middle of the floor generating a smothering heat. The place smelled like stale urine, fresh feces, musty clothing, and unwashed human bodies. The odor was so strong that Doc could taste it, had to acknowledge it with every breath.

BJ was lying on a blanket facing away from the stove. He was pale, thin, his ribs visible through his ragged T-shirt. He shivered continuously. Doc knew without asking that BJ had been having one watery bowel movement after another, that he was too weak to get to the outhouse, too sick to know that he was lying in his own excrement. Doc rolled him gently onto his back. BJ stared straight up, not because he was looking, but because that was the way his head was facing. With his free hand, Doc captured the antique stethoscope that swung around his neck and placed it on the boy's skeletal chest. The heart sounds were distant and rapid. There were crackles in both lungs; Doc knew they were full of mucous and pus. He traced needle tracks on BJ's forearms with his index finger, wondered who had taught this man with a child's mind how to use drugs, what favors he had then exchanged to feed such an appetite. He pinched the loose skin on BJ's belly.

"He needs to go to the hospital, Burl. He's dehydrated, and he has pneumonia in both lungs." He knew Burl's answer even before he said the words.

"Hell, Doc, it's just a case of the trots. Just treat 'em like you'd treat one 'a your downtown patients. I ain't no doctor, but I figger you got a bottle of sugar water out in that new Jeep of yours. Put a needle in his arm, give him some 'a that. Put a plug of penicillin in his ass. He'll be OK in the mornin'. Hell, you know I'm good for it, if that's what you're worried about. If he was that sick, I'd already took him to the hospital."

Doc bit his lip, turned to Burl. "This is not just a case of the 'trots'. It's far more serious than that. I don't have the expertise to manage this." His lip curled in spite of his effort to control it. "And neither do you."

Burl sputtered, wiped his nose, then jammed his hands behind the bib of his overalls while he paced around the room. Jan stood docile as a milk cow, gumming her tobacco, saying nothing.

"Can't you just do something for him here, Doc?" Burl asked, his voice taking on a persecuted tone. "We can't get to Knoxville. My truck...neither one of us is fit to drive, anyhow."

Doc sighed. *These two should have smothered under the weight of their own ignorance decades ago.* "I'll go over to the Crabtree's and call the ambulance. Don't touch BJ while I'm gone," he warned over his shoulder, like there was any danger of it. "I'll be back," he yelled from the yard, just for emphasis. "Boil some water while I'm gone."

He returned in less than thirty minutes to find that Burl had paced the whole time and Jan hadn't moved. They hadn't boiled the water, either, so Doc had to do that before he could clean BJ and dress him in a pair of flannel pajamas that Mrs. Crabtree had donated. Burl watched, muttered, and wrung his hands. Jan stared out the window or at Doc or Burl, but never at BJ. From time to time, she spit into a filthy Dixie cup.

Doc heard the ambulance moaning in the distance. He followed its progress by the sound until it appeared in the yard, blue lights flashing, short-wave radio crackling meaningless phrases into the cold night air. He went outside to meet the paramedics and lead them to BJ.

There were two of them, both young, one of them a woman.

"Be careful," Doc said. "Best I can tell, he was being treated for AIDS."

"Everyone's contagious anymore, Doc," the woman said as she pulled on a pair of disposable rubber gloves. "We're careful with everybody."

Doc stepped back as the paramedics rolled the gurney out the door, watched as they slid the stretcher through the ambulance doors. BJ twisted slowly to his side, moved his knees toward his chest, roused a little, and seemed to focus on Doc for an instant before his eyes glazed over again. Doc remembered the rueful baby smile from twenty-five years before.

He turned to Burl who squatted on the porch, smoking a cigarette, alternately appearing then disappearing as the emergency lights on the ambulance flashed over him in a rhythm as regular as a heartbeat. Behind him, Jan's silhouette on the window shade occasionally dipped its head to spit. The siren wailed long after the ambulance was out of sight.

RUNAWAY

Mom wouldn't of liked it if she knew the judge had sent me to live with her sister. She always said Harriet was trashy. I come to live with her in a tarpaper shack, set in the bend of one of the curves that hooks together to make up highway 70. Railroad tracks run along the bank behind it, squeezing the house into the bend of the road. The gravel shoulder of the highway made most of our front yard.

The house didn't have no front porch. Felix, the man Harriet stayed with, laid planks across some cinder blocks for us to use as steps. The tin roof had rusted out in a few spots. I slept in the attic, so I got to know the leaky parts of that roof pretty well. A wood-burning stove, downstairs, kept the house smoky, smelly and not very warm.

Mom and I never associated with Harriet. Harriet had quit school in the tenth grade to live with a man a lot older than her. There had been a lot of men since then, too, according to Mom. I reckon that's why Mom called her trash.

They weren't no men in my mom's life, except me. She said my dad was killed in the war, but she never said which one. Mom died right after I turned fourteen. I come home from school and found her sitting in the bathtub with both her wrists slit clear to the bone, the last drops of her blood circling down the drain. After that, Doc Haskins tried to get me into foster care. He was old by then, an' wore out, so he might not have tried as hard as he could've. I reckon the judge didn't have much choice but to send me to Harriet's. He fixed it so the state would send her a check every month for taking care of me, so she was willing. Besides, I had no other kin.

Harriet used to be pretty. When I moved in, she looked a lot older than thirty-six. Her bleached blonde hair still hung down around her shoulders like it did when she dropped out of high school. She wore loose baggy clothes to hide the weight she had gained. When she talked her hand automatically flipped up to cover her bad teeth.

She had lived with Felix longer than any of her other men. I don't think it was because she loved him the most, though. I think it would of been awful hard for her to leave unless he had wanted her to go. He had a bald head, slick and shiny, that pulled his eyes back tight, like a snake's. His arms stayed hard as ax handles, without any exercise that I ever saw. His right arm had a tattoo of a naked woman, lounging with her head on his shoulder, and her bare feet propped on his elbow. Thick curly hair crept out at the neck of his sleeveless undershirt. I think Harriet was 'fraid of him. He sure scared me.

Felix nor Harriet paid any mind to me. They stayed occupied with each other. Harriet wore a bathrobe around the house all the time, usually without a stitch on underneath it. If she walked by Felix, he would smack her across her bottom and tell her she had a butt like a Perch'n mare. If he walked by her, he'd stick his hand under her robe and rub at her breast. Either way, she'd giggle. He'd look as proud as if he had just discovered fire.

I think with me around, Felix saw some value in having kids. I remember him talking to Harriet about how they could use some extra money. That's how I first figured out they was getting money for me. They always quit talking when I come in earshot, but Harriet didn't seem too happy with the idea.

Felix won out, 'cause they finally made an appointment with the lady at the Department of Human Services for Marion County. Felix covered his tattoo with a wrinkled, long sleeve shirt. Harriet posed as a childless mother.

They must of been pretty convincing. The social worker called them back a week later to tell them about Maggie. She told Felix that Maggie was in the Juvenile Center in Nashville. She hadn't done nothing bad. She just didn't have no place to go. I could tell by the way he talked that Felix was excited. Then at the last minute, his face turned dark and the veins in his forehead started to bulge out, real prominent. Me and Harriet set on the couch and watched Felix cover the phone with his hand, and cuss under his breath. He told the social worker that he'd have to call her back. He needed to think before he took on the responsibility of a handicapped child. He hung up the phone and started pacing around the room, calling Maggie a deaf mute, the same way you'd talk about tainted meat. He stormed outside, still cussing.

We heard the engine in his old station wagon rev real loud, then fade out as he headed down the road toward the Highway 70 tavern. Harriet told me that that's where he went when he needed to think. When he come back, he had calmed down a lot. First thing next morning, he called the lady back, and told her he and Harriet would do their best for Maggie. They packed the car and headed for Nashville that same day.

I stayed home and waited. Every hour, from the time they left, I either looked out the window, or stood on the wobbly front steps, listening for Felix's old station wagon with its gutted mufflers. I was as excited as if we was expecting a newborn. They was late getting home; eight hours later than I calculated it would take. Felix pulled off the highway and parked next to the woodpile. He and Harriet rolled out of the car and went in the house leaning on each other and laughing. I could tell by how they acted that they had stopped somewhere to celebrate.

Maggie set in the back of the car, looking real vulnerable. I knew how she looked, even then, but I didn't know the word for it till years later. For a while, when I was thinking about trying to get my high school equivalency diploma, I memorized word definitions. I tried to learn a new word every day. One day, when I come across that word, vulnerable, I just 'membered Maggie, in that car, that day.

I was struck on her that first time I seen her. Her shiny black hair curled off her head into a long thick ponytail. She had dark skin like she had a suntan even in the middle of winter. Her eyes drawed me to her. They were big, wide and brown. Them sad eyes made me feel like she needed looking after.

I helped Maggie carry her stuff up into the attic with mine. They's no stairs. We had to climb a ladder to get up there. I made a trip with her stuff, then I come back down to get her.

She crawled up into the attic, an' stood up, looking around her. They's only two old mattresses, flat on the floor, with blankets folded on top of them. I put Maggie's suitcase on the one next to a tiny window. I think I could see a thank you just underneath the brown in her eyes. She started to unpack her things. All of a sudden, her head jerked up an' she cocked her ear toward the window. I watched her eyes, and I imagined I saw question marks. She walked over and opened the window with a far-off expression on her face. I could barely hear a train whistling. The blowing got louder and louder as the train busted across the open area just behind the house.

I just set, studying Maggie. She didn't look like she was fourteen. And, she could hear pretty good for somebody who's supposed to be deaf. I wondered if she could talk and just didn't.

Harriet hollered up the ladder for me to come down and carry in some wood. We both come down, Maggie first, then me. Felix stood at the bottom like he was going to help her. I don't know why it surprised me when I caught him looking up her dress. I looked down right into his snake eyes, and he just glared back at me. I put so much wood in that stove that the door glowed red with the heat of it.

We set down to supper at the flimsy card table circled with metal folding chairs. Me and Maggie ate pinto beans and corn bread on saucers that didn't match. Maggie ate hers holding her fork real proper, with her left hand in her lap. She chewed slow and looked straight at her plate. Someone had taught her some manners.

I could tell Felix was getting mad. He didn't like uppity people or uppity ways. He kept chewing and looking real hard at Maggie. She finished her food and laid her fork down on the edge of her plate. Felix put down his spoon and felt in his shirt for a cigarette. He scraped his chair back and burped real loud. Maggie didn't look at him. He dipped his hand in Harriet's bathrobe and kept looking at Maggie. She avoided his eyes.

Finally, he moved over to his rented television set. While he cussed at the picture and worked with the rabbit ears, me and Maggie started to pick up the plates. We had the place cleaned, lickety split. Soon's we finished, I motioned for Maggie to get her coat. I had learned not to ask Felix or Harriet if I could go out. They always said no. If I just left, they never said nothing less the fire burned down. They'd walk five miles to tell me to carry in a stick of wood. I figured they'd do for a while, the way I had stoked that fire before supper.

Me and Maggie snuck out the back door an' run down the steps into the gravel. It surprised me when she reached out an' took hold of my hand. Just like that, I had somebody who depended on me. I led her up the bank toward the tracks. She looked both directions, then she stepped up on the near one. She motioned me to do the same, then she held her finger across her lips. I could feel a real faint vibration under my feet. I looked down at the rail. I couldn't see it move at all.

She took my hand again and led me away from the tracks. She looked like she was waiting for something. After a few minutes, we heard another train whistle blowing. Pretty soon the train itself come into sight. We stood there while it blew by us, bending the tracks with its weight, and shaking the ground underneath us, blowing Maggie's hair around her face. I felt Maggie take hold of my hand again. She almost looked happy.

We walked back to the house in the dark. I looked through the glass in the kitchen door. Felix and Harriet was still involved with each other and their television program, so we sat on the back steps in the cold. I told Maggie how Felix scared me and how my mom called Harriet trash. I told her how they didn't let me go to school, even though I was supposed to be in the ninth grade. I showed her my notebook, where I wrote stuff down, to remember. Before I knew it, I even told her that I had a hideout and that I planned to run away. She looked at me again, full in the face, worried. I think she almost talked.

We finally snuck back in through the back door, climbed the ladder to the attic and got in our beds. I must've went to sleep pretty quick. I remember a flashlight shining round and round the room, waking me and blinding me at the same time. The cutting edge of the light settled on Maggie before the room went dark again. My mind stayed fuzzy like I was partly still dreaming. I ain't ashamed to tell you, I was scared.

I sensed Felix pull his bulk into the attic. I felt the floor strain under him as he made his way toward Maggie's cot. A strand of moonlight shined in through the window over her bed. I could see him when he set down on the edge of her mattress an' folded back her blankets.

The light must of woke Maggie up too. Soon as he set down, she fought him like a trapped animal. He cussed her, out loud. He didn't care if I heard him or not. He knew I couldn't of stopped him anyway. I could see her eyes, plain, in the moonlight. She'd struggle with him, then she'd look toward me like she's wondering what I'm waiting for. Then, she'd fight some more. My body wouldn't move, no matter what I told it to do. I felt exactly like one of them dreams where you want to run from something terrible, but everything that needs to happen to save you happens in slow motion.

I watched Felix lay his body over hers, smothering her under his weight. Then, all of a sudden, her eyes opened real wide, like she's surprised and hurting at the same time. He had her body pinned against the mattress, but she could still roll her head, back and forth, hard, so that it banged against the wall over and over. Her mouth stayed open, like somebody who's screaming, but she didn't make a sound. She quit looking for me.

Finally, I seen Felix stand part way and hitch up his britches. He walked stooped over so his head wouldn't hit the ceiling. Before he stepped on the ladder, he turned back, looked toward me and spit. I felt my britches turn warm where my bladder let go.

I heard Maggie sniffing after he crawled down the ladder. When I got my muscles to where they'd work again, I crawled over to her. She had pulled her blanket up to her chin and rolled her body to face toward the wall. I reached for her hand, but she pulled away, real sharp. I was so ashamed, I thought I would bust. I set next to her the rest of the night, miserable, wet and crying.

The next morning, Felix took Harriet and went somewhere till way up in the afternoon. They come back, laughing and pinching at each other, smelling like beer and cigarette smoke. Me and Maggie went outside soon as they come home. Maggie set down on a cinder block at the corner of the house, while I made out like I was trying to throw rocks clean across the highway. I tried not to let on that I was watching her. She caught me looking, once, and rubbed her eyes hard with the back of her hand. She stood back up, an' I could tell it hurt her.

We sat through another supper of beans and bread. Felix ignored us, scooping his food on a spoon with his thumb. Harriet giggled and tried to hold her fork like Maggie. Maggie didn't eat hardly nothing. She went straight to the attic as soon as Felix left the table. I cleaned the dishes by myself.

It was dark when I finished. I walked out by myself and stood on the railroad track. I felt a train coming but I still just stood there, trying to call back the good feelings I had when Maggie stood there with me. I could hear the train bearing down on me. It got close enough that I could see the panic in the engineer's eyes, while he tried to blow me off the tracks with his whistle. I stepped off at the last fraction of a second. I snuck back into the house, and went up to the attic, like I meant to go to bed.

I found Maggie setting on the edge of my bed with her suitcase packed. I didn't say nothing. I just put my extra jeans and shirt in a sack with the Barlow knife that Felix thought he'd lost. I put my stuff down next to her suitcase.

Maggie didn't move. I squatted down next to her and put my hand on hers. She didn't pull back. She looked at me and there ain't no question marks in her eyes this time. She squeezed my hand a little. We set there till we heard Felix and Harriet settle into bed.

When they both started snoring, I crawled over to the edge of the ladder, where I could see them. Then, I crawled down with my sack of clothes, tiptoed to the back door, and dropped it on the steps. The Barlow made a loud clunk on the wood. Felix and Harriet kept on snoring. I

climbed back up the ladder. Maggie handed me her suitcase. I helped her down again, real careful. I could tell she
hurt. Last, I took some bread off the stove, and wrapped it
with some canned fruit and a box of matches. I dropped it
all in the sack with my britches. I figured when we got to
my hideout, I could build us a fire and Maggie might feel
like eating a little.

I took her hand and pulled her up the bank. We lit
out walking along the middle of the tracks toward the east.
The moon shined cold and bright so we could see down the
tracks for nearly a mile. That worried me 'cause we could
be seen just as easy. I wanted to get settled before Maggie
gave out on me. I knowed she couldn't walk through the
woods, the way she hurt.

We walked about an hour before we come to the
place where the railroad tracks shot out over empty air. More
than once during the daytime, I'd walked out along that trestle toward the other side of the gorge. I'd never gone beyond
halfway. I don't know why. I just always stopped. Lots of
times, I'd sit an' dangle my legs over the side, a hundred feet
above the ribbon of water that wiggled along the bottom of
the ravine. That's how I found my cave. I was setting looking
back toward where I'd been, and I seen the mouth of it, partly hid by the bushes. You couldn't see it looking down from
the near edge 'cause it nestled back under the bluff.

Somebody had used it years before, because I found
a path all growed up, leading down to it. After I had it
cleaned out, I started stealing stuff from Harriet and Felix.
I only took a little at a time, but I had a pretty good stockpile now. I hadn't ever told myself that I'd run away before
I told it to Maggie. I reckon part of me knew it.

I set our stuff on the ground and told Maggie she'd
need to hold on to me. I didn't tell her it's almost straight
down, if we fell. I could tell I scared her by the way her hand
got real stiff and sweaty. I decided to go down first, then

come back up, just to show her how easy it was. I crawled down the bank, an' pulled into the mouth of the cave. The blankets an' stuff I had stored back there felt warm an' dry. I felt like we was setting up housekeeping. I knew I could take care of Maggie. I just needed another chance.

I scrambled back up the path to get Maggie. I couldn't of been gone more than five minutes. Just like that, she was gone. I looked in every direction possible before I looked at the trestle. I knew that's where she went, even while I looked the other ways. Finally, I picked out her shadow, about mid-ways across, walking real slow. All of a sudden, I seen her freeze in the middle of the tracks. Her head jerked up, quick, like something had took her attention away from where she had been watching each step real careful. I reckon she must of felt some vibrations. She looked back and forth real fast, like she was judging her chances of making it to one side or the other. Then, she set her suitcase on the tracks beside her.

Before I could see it, I barely heard the noise of a train across the ravine. The engine was the same gray black as the night, so for a moment, it looked like the headlight on the front of it was moving on its own, not attached to anything. The front edge of the light jerked and bobbed fifty yards in front of the train. The whistle blared from the invisible engine behind it. When the light first touched Maggie, it looked like that's what pushed her over the edge.

She fell in slow motion. She didn't flail her arms or legs. Her shadow turned slowly round and round like a helicopter blade. She fell with as much dignity as when she set down to supper with us. I watched her disappear into the pitch-black darkness. The metal wheels of the train sliced her cardboard suitcase open on the tracks, scattering her belongings into the treetops below. When I come to myself, I was walking along that trestle with my mouth open wide, like I was screaming. I couldn't hear a sound.

What Noma Meant to Say

Noma Gentry leaned on her walker and stared out the picture window overlooking the lawn circling Shannondale like a moat. She squinted her eyes, hunched her shoulders, and bent her knees a little, as if searching a half century of horizons back to the gray morning when she watched Hiram back the hay wagon into the barn for the last time.

She had never understood why he continued to work so hard, even after they couldn't pretend to own the farm. The week prior, they'd stood on the sidewalk in front of the First National Bank of Oak Grove and watched little clouds form where their warm breath collided with cold December air. Hiram picked at imaginary flaws in the floppy brim of the straw hat he'd worn for years to protect him from the relentless glare of the sun. At the last minute, he'd shrugged a brown dress coat over his bib overalls, all that was left of the suit he'd worn to marry Noma. She wore her apron over her work dress. The laces wrapped twice around her waist and ending in a large, looping bowknot on her stomach. Their two boys, too young to understand grinding poverty but old enough to sense the gravity of this situation, stood in the seat of the truck, and watched.

Sweat glistened on Hiram's upper lip.

"He's just a man," Noma said.

"I'll just talk to him," Hiram said, like it was an idea that had just occurred to him.

They'd sat in the dark that last morning and drank scalding black coffee. She savored their early morning ruminations, sometimes because of the things they left unsaid, not talking about Russian missiles in Cuba or the Mark of the Beast or, on that morning, the impending foreclosure on the farm that had been in his family since before the Civil War.

His voice split the silence. "I love you," he had said.

The words hung in the air over the kitchen table as if they had just appeared, unconnected to a human thought. Hiram rationed his words, as if the supply was limited and he feared he'd use his allotment before running out of things to say. He never said "I love you" to Noma in the daylight. He never failed to say it at bedtime. Noma always answered, reassured that the last thing that either of them heard before they slept every evening was a private, renewal of their wedding vows, to love each other, for better or worse. She looked out the kitchen window, sipping the coffee he always made too strong.

"I love you, too," she said.

She waited for Hiram to finish loading hay bales out of the loft, then pull the wagon into the pasture to feed their few remaining cows. She'd seen him step off the wagon bed a thousand other times, letting his knees and hips absorb the impact of the drop without jarring, the way she imagined he did when he was a paratrooper in WWII. The wind puffed again, cold, straight from the north, moaning a little around the corner of the house. His body seemed to float, then turn slowly, almost gracefully toward her. His head bowed at an awkward angle. His arms hung limp at his side. She realized that what he meant to say that morning was "Goodbye."

The nurse appeared out of nowhere. "Need to rest?" she asked. She moved a chair behind Noma to where it just touched the back of her legs.

"Poor little thing," Noma answered, using half of her working vocabulary. Until a few months ago, she could still say her birthday, but just like the ignition on Hiram's pick-up truck that had to grind and grind until the starter caught and the motor roared into life, she had to peck her fingertips on the table-top and say "twenty-two" over and over until finally "Twenty-two October nineteen-oh-nine" erupted. She said it in a distinctive rhythm, as if the cadence was as much a part of the memory as the date.

Noma rocked back and forth slightly, as if her body, like her mind, teetered between the things she couldn't remember and the ones she couldn't forget. The walker slipped. Noma plunked down hard on the chair.

"Are you OK?" asked the nurse.

"Bless its heart," Noma answered.

The nurse adjusted Noma's robe and said something else that Noma didn't hear because she was already engrossed in a blue jay that flew onto and off the bird bath outside the window while a well-fed tabby cat lashed its tail and skulked nearby.

"Bless its heart," she said as if she felt sorry for the bird. "Poor little thing."

There were a half dozen other Shannondale patients in the day room. They had paid no attention to Noma and her leaning, squatting and muttering over her walker. They wandered in their own forests. Like Noma, they had skirted around the edges for years, going through the motions of normalcy, breathing, eating, working, sleeping, thinking that Truman was president and not Clinton or that it was May instead of September or fall instead of spring.

Noma had walked deep into her personal forest never to return the night she called the Oak Grove police to report that dope addicts had taken residence in the crawl space under her house. The young officer had walked with her from room to room, clicked on lights, checked in closets, and looked under furniture. He went outside and aimed his flashlight into the trees, at the shrubbery, between the steps, and under the porch.

"I'm not finding anything, Mrs. Gentry," he said.

Each person in the dayroom had their unique travel log chronicling a journey from independence to dependence, from insight to oblivion, from hiding around the edges of the deep dark woods to becoming eternally lost inside it. Every patient had a child who finally shrugged in defeat, then moved their mother or father to a place where an imaginary world could expand safely in a semi-private room, where marriages that had spanned half a century ended as a stranger's face in a black and white photograph on a cheap bedside table.

The day nurse turned to the other patients.

"Good afternoon," she said.

Rheumy eyes looked toward her. No one answered.

She turned the radio on and adjusted the volume. A preacher at WOAK finished his Sunday afternoon sermon about escaping the wrath to come. Organ music played the melody to "Farther Along," while the disc jockey read the weekly obituary and extolled the virtues of a pre-paid funeral plan from Tauscher's mortuary.

A quiet and aloof former schoolteacher pursed her lips like an asterisk, extended her gnarled index finger and marked out the rhythm for a classroom full of unruly students that still lived in her mind. The other residents leaned over their wheelchair armrests or tilted forward against their chest restraints, frozen in waxy postures, gazing with empty eyes into a future they no longer feared.

Noma nodded her head slightly as if a memory of the music was trying to wriggle free from the plaques and tangles that held it submerged. Before her last stroke cauterized the speech area of her brain, she shuffled the halls and sang, "Some glad morning, when this life is ov-er, I'll... fly away." Sometimes, a burly man with a phlegmy cough echoed the bass refrain from down the hall, "in the morning." After he died, she lowered her voice and sang it herself.

Noma rocked, slowly gathering momentum to stand again.

The nurse put her hand on the cross bar to steady the walker. "Tired of sittin' already?" she asked. For a moment, their hands were side by side, Noma's with fingers that twisted at each joint and translucent skin that showed her veins like a relief map, and the nurse's smooth, symmetric, and tan.

"Bless… its…heart," Noma said, punctuating each rocking motion with a word to add momentum. "Poor… lit…tle… thing," she continued.

She bent over with her elbows on her walker and rested for a minute. Then she stood and leaned a little to the left so her right foot could scoot on the tile, a gait she'd acquired gradually after a stroke weakened the right half of her body.

Years earlier, before the doors to D-wing were set with alarms and before Noma needed assistance, she had wandered off the campus and ambled down the one mile stretch of highway into town. The nurses and aides searched all over Shannodale until someone called from Bill's Meat Market where she had loaded a grocery cart and was chatting with the cashier at the register about her growing boy's appetite and how she enjoyed her new job at the hosiery mill. She couldn't remember either of her boys' names by then. Her mind held a composite of the two, one generic son that she inserted into whatever distorted recollection she might have.

Noma turned in a series of fragmented steps to follow the nurse. She winced when either foot accepted her full weight. She shuffled a few steps, scooting her walker in front of her, then rested and watched as the nurse stopped beside a man with a string of drool that stretched from his sagging lower lip to a moist spot on his plaid flannel shirt. He bore little resemblance to the boy who'd hitchhiked to the Navy Recruiting station in Knoxville the day after he graduated from Oak Grove High school in 1943, anxious that the war would stop without him. The nurse wiped his mouth with a paper towel, then uncapped the tube that entered through his abdominal wall and ended in his stomach. She poured an elixir of medicines that were as pointless as his mind was blank.

They moved to the next patient, a former deacon at the First Baptist Church. His daughter brought him to live at Shannondale when she found him living in squalid conditions in the home where she grew up. He rarely spoke, except to pray long prayers, using flowery lines and beautiful words when called upon to deliver the blessing for the evening meal.

"Take your time," the nurse said as she took colored pills of different sizes and shapes and placed them in his mouth. "Now, take a sip of water." She waited for him to swallow. "Now stick out your tongue," she said. She peered inside to make sure all the pills were gone.

They moved from one patient to the next. The nurse placed pills and sips of water onto the desiccated tongues of people whose personalities had disappeared with their memories and left no distinctive features other than the typewritten name and birthdates on their plastic wristbands. Noma scooted along behind like an acolyte.

"Poor little thing," she said.

May you swallow and not get choked.

May the good Lord bless and keep you....

"Bless its heart."

They stopped before a cadaverous old man who sat propped in his Geri-chair. His back was curved so that his neck had to be buttressed on pillows. People joked that he had developed his deformity from years of hunching over, counting his money. An oil painting, commissioned by his mother when he was young and his body arrow straight, still hung on the wall in First National Bank lobby.

The nurse fluffed a pillow under the banker's neck. She adjusted his hands on his belly, one over the other, to look like he meant them to be there. The broad blue veins glistened like ribbons through his cadaver-white skin. She placed a pill on his tongue. A weak, wet cough interrupted his shallow breathing.

"Poor little thing," Noma said.

"He's pitiful, ain't he?" the nurse said. "They say he used to be rich."

Noma gently ran the tip of her arthritic finger along the bones of the banker's forehead where the fat had melted away and the skin stretched tight over his skull. A blind person might have performed the same gentle gesture in an effort to recognize a loved one they couldn't see.

The nurse put a thick yellow slurry of medicine into a little plastic cup and dribbled it into his mouth. She watched him swallow, then helped him settle back onto his pillow. She penciled her note, then pushed her cart toward the door and disappeared down the hall.

Noma frowned again, as if she had recognized the outline of the man from that morning decades past when he hunched over his mahogany desk and wrote on a sheet of paper the dollar amount that Hiram would need to pay just to postpone losing the farm for another year. He had pushed it toward them with the eraser end of his pencil, as if by not touching it, he somehow absolved himself of his part in the destruction of the hopes and dreams they'd planted there.

The banker sputtered and coughed. His mouth opened and closed like a baby bird. His eyes bulged, watered, and gave a reflexive frantic unseeing look around the room, then rolled back under his wispy white eyebrows and closed like he was asleep. A white froth gathered in the corner of his mouth. His lips turned as blue as the veins in the back of his hands. The room filled with a feculent odor as his sphincter muscles relaxed.

Noma turned to the window. The winter sun had just dropped behind Roan Mountain leaving only the frowning silhouette of the ridgeline on the horizon. A red light blinked at the top of the WOAK radio antenna perched high on the top of the fire tower warning the occasional low flying aircraft to stay clear. She leaned on her walker unencumbered by the fading wake of painful memories or the fear of eternity.

"Poor little thing," she said. "Bless its heart."

THE VEIL

Doc Haskins watched through the kitchen window as the sun skimmed westward across the top of Roan Mountain. The trip to Knoxville was tiring and traumatic, too much for old folks to manage in one day. They were still sweaty from the July heat and a little carsick from the ride, but he had insisted that Lorrie try to eat something as soon as they were home. She had picked at her breakfast hours earlier and hadn't had a bite since.

Lorrie pushed her bowl away, jostling a dollop of stew onto the Irish linen tablecloth. "I can't," she said. She checked the white polka dots on her navy blue dress for splatters, like it was an afterthought, then fingered the pearl necklace Doc bought her years ago. "I'm just not hungry." She stood, started to pick up the dishes.

Doc let his soup trickle off the spoon and dribble back into the bowl. "I'll clean up," he said. He put one of Lorrie's aprons on over his brown suit, then opened, gently slammed, then reopened cabinet doors while he searched for dish detergent. Lorrie retreated to the living room to her rocking chair, to her books.

She had seemed ill at ease with the university doctor. *Who wouldn't? He was young enough to be our grandson, but he was so arrogant.* Doc didn't expect anything extra, but it galled him a little to hear the doctor call his wife Lorrie instead of Mrs. Haskins.

She seemed reluctant to let him examine her. She appeared doubtful, too, when he claimed to feel a "fullness" deep in the pit of her stomach. He recommended that she see a cancer specialist, predicted that she would certainly need chemotherapy and probably "a little cobalt."

"That sounds bad," Lorrie said.

"There's no such thing as a 'good' cancer," the doctor agreed, nodding grimly, like he was the new sheriff in town. "But you must keep a positive attitude so you can fight it."

Doc recalled Lorrie's image as he helped her don the examination gown. Her backbone looked like knots tied in baling twine. Her skin sagged in loose wrinkles from her weight loss. She wasn't up to much of a fight.

"Even if the treatment doesn't help, Lorrie," he continued, "the information we gather might help your children or your grandchildren someday."

It was a stock phrase, one that all doctors say, one that sounds profound but isn't. Doc Haskins had used it himself in his small-town general practice. He felt Lorrie shrink against his arm like something inside her was leaking out.

Doc finished washing the dishes, wiped the table, then draped the apron over a kitchen chair and joined Lorrie in the living room. He loosened his bow tie, unbuttoned his collar, settled in his overstuffed recliner with a pile of unread medical journals stacked on either side.

"I don't see the point," she said.

Was the break in her voice from emotion or fatigue?

"If I don't take the treatment, I die," she said. "If I do take it, you drive me back and forth to Knoxville for a few weeks for some treatment that will make me sicker, and I die anyway."

His craggy face, furrowed as deep as the farmland surrounding Oak Grove, tried to rearrange itself into a smile.

"We're all going to die," he said. "But we don't have to just give in to it." It was another stock answer, one he regretted as soon as he heard the words leave his mouth.

She rubbed his big, knobby fingers with her tiny, chalk-white hand, a latticework of blue veins visible just under her skin. "How did you suture with your knuckles this way?" she asked. He once could repair the tiniest cut on the vermillion border of a wrestling child's lip and leave only the hint of a scar.

"I don't know," he said. "Practice, I guess. Doing the same thing over and over."

They sat without speaking, her occasional gentle squeeze on his hand the only reminder that she was still thinking, still formulating words in her mind, arranging her thoughts.

"Promise me that you won't let me hurt," she said. She rubbed Doc's hand, as if to remind him that she knew there was more to him than showed on the outside. "These young doctors don't know there's a difference in living longer and dying slower."

It was a warm afternoon, but Lorrie insisted that Doc wrap her feet and legs in a blanket, drape a shawl across her shoulders, and push her wheelchair to the oak tree in their backyard. They had spent the morning looking at photographs from her summertime travels. He imagined her showing these same pictures to her students, offering them her documentary of other people and far-off places as proof that there was a world beyond the Oak Grove city limits.

"This was my favorite place to wait for you to come home," she said. "I've sat here and read for hours."

It wasn't an accusation, but it felt like one.

"I always thought of you when I read Chekhov," she continued. She had a faraway look in her eyes. "Medicine was his mistress, too."

Mistress? That seems a little harsh.

She reached for his hand without looking at him, as if she could hear his thoughts. "Did you miss me when I traveled all those summers?" she asked.

After their son Zade died, Doc encouraged Lorrie to travel. He wanted her to stay busy, to keep her mind occupied. He immersed himself in his practice, refused to be away from Oak Grove more than a night or two at a time until he was nearly sixty.

"It was like lancing a boil," he said. "Sometimes necessary. Never desirable."

A breeze rustled through the leaves above them. Lorrie craned her head back where she could look up at the tree. "I used to look into those branches and imagine how Michelangelo felt, lying on his back, painting the ceiling of the Sistine Chapel."

Doc looked up. The leaves had changed from green to gold to russet since their trip to the university hospital. He didn't see the ceiling of a chapel. He couldn't imagine how Michelangelo felt. He needed to find out more about Dr. Chekhov, too.

Lorrie reversed her days and nights, blended her memory with her imagination, saw things that were not real, and didn't see things that were. He had to move her rocking chair from the living room and replace it with a hospital bed. She wet herself. He changed her. She vomited. He cleaned her. She hurt. He pinched the skin on her belly and injected morphine.

Her eyes turned a deep orange. Her hands swelled so quickly Doc could barely soap her wedding band off. Her urine turned the same coffee color as the winter leaves on the ground under the oak tree. Her breath took on a sweet odor, one that didn't fade no matter how often or how thoroughly he cleaned her mouth.

"Don't look at me," Lorrie said when she caught him studying her. "I don't like it."

Sometimes she woke and asked questions from nowhere, like she was dreaming a discussion, and when she roused, just continued the conversation.

"What do you think will happen after I die?" she asked.

"I don't know," he said. "I'll..." He wanted to tell her that he hadn't been able to imagine life without her.

"Do you think there is a place we go, to another life?" she asked. She closed her eyes again, seemed to sleep.

Doc believed death was a biologic fact, the outer boundary to life, that in the universe there is no change in the quantity of matter, only in the form that matter takes; ashes to ashes, dust to dust. That's all we are. That's all we become.

"A doctor in one of Faulkner's novels said that death only exists in the minds of the survivors, that the actual death is no more significant than a tenant changing tenements," she said, as if he had answered her.

Doc scanned her bookshelves, wondered which book she referenced.

"What do *you* think?" he asked, helplessly pushing the point, dreading her answer. "Do you think there is a place we go to after we die?"

"Oh, yes," she said. "I talk to people who are there. They're waiting for me."

"Who?" he asked, arching his eyebrow. He had always said it was best to humor a delirious patient. Say what they need to hear. Ask what they want to answer. "Who have you talked to?"

"Family," she said.

Doc's mind strayed helplessly to the memory of their son.

"My daddy visited me one night. He didn't say anything, just stood at the edge of my bed and shimmered in and out of the light. He was wearing the suit we buried him in, except he was wearing his hat. I closed my eyes, and when I opened them, he was gone. I thought it was a dream."

"It was," Doc said. He sounded harsh, even to himself. "Maybe, it was," he repeated in a softer voice, hoping she hadn't heard him the first time.

"Maybe. But I never had it before. And if it was a dream, I would have been afraid," she said. "I was glad to see him. I felt safe."

"Have you seen anyone else?"

"Sometimes I see Mom. My brother was standing behind her once." Lorrie's mother died in her sleep decades earlier. Her only brother died in France, during the war. "I guess they're trying to reassure me."

Doc pinched the bridge of his nose, squinted his eyelids tight. He had heard hundreds of tearful stories about death visitations, accepted them as signs of hysteria or emotional incompetence. He had resisted sarcasm, patted slumped shoulders, and said things like, "There now, he's in a better place." He had said these words without feeling them, done these things without believing them, over and over. It was part of the role, part of being a small-town doctor.

"So where do you think they are traveling from?" he asked. "And why was your dad still wearing his burial suit? Don't you think it's because that was your last memory of him?"

"I don't know," she answered. "Next time I'll ask."

She said it like their whole conversation was rational, logical, like she knew and he accepted that there was a thin veil separating the dead from the living, one that people could step through, then step back again, at their pleasure, from wherever they are to wherever this is.

She expected there to be a next time.

It was January, bitter cold. Doc had left Lorrie asleep to stand in the darkness on the back porch and cough the stagnant air from his lungs. When he returned, he found

Zade sitting on the piano bench, facing the window, looking away from Doc. It was almost as surprising that he was at the piano as it was that he was even present. Lorrie had hopes that she could mold him into a cultured little boy, had tried to teach him piano before he started school, and had insisted that he practice a few minutes every day. Zade resisted, much preferring to be in the dirt, kicking a ball, climbing a tree, doing little boy things. Even now, he wore the striped T-shirt, the muddy jeans, the US Keds tennis shoes with one of them unlaced, the uniform of all Oak Grove first graders in the 1960s.

Doc tried to position himself where he could see Zade's face. He wanted to touch the tiny bruise on the boy's forehead, still wanted to understand how a fall from a playground sliding board could cause such a trivial appearing wound yet still be fatal. The room seemed to swivel so that no matter how he approached, his only view was the skinny neck, the narrow shoulders, and the perfect symmetry of the round little head with the little boy buzz cut. That much hadn't changed in thirty-five years.

Memories that had haunted him—images that had roused him from sleep and left him sitting on his bedside with a pounding heart and sweaty palms—played like a movie in his mind once more. He saw Zade's mouth make a perfect circle, watched his head turn toward him with his eyes already glazed over, saw his face soften, heard him exhale a soft whooshing sound like he was blowing out a birthday candle. He remembered how Lorrie perched on a stainless-steel exam stool and rocked her body back and forth, how she cried in a high-pitched moan that didn't stop even when she took a breath, how she rebuffed Doc's attempt to comfort himself by holding her. He pictured their pastor in his shiny shoes and cheap suit, heard again his empty prayer that mentioned faith smaller than a mustard seed and mountains to be moved, recalled the way he held both Lorrie's hands in his never calloused ones and told her, "God just let us borrow Zade for a while. He took him back to be with Him."

Lorrie roused, mumbled something. Her breathing changed from quiet and shallow to deep and rapid. Her eyes searched the room, frantic, until they settled on Doc. He leaned over her, put ice chips on her tongue, considered another dose of morphine, then adjusted the moist washcloth on her forehead.

"Zade is here," Doc said, thinking that might calm her. "It's Zade."

She locked her gaze on Doc, magnetized him so that he couldn't look away. Her wide, blue eyes were like mirrors in which he saw his reflection staring back; a tired old man with a halo of white hair growing directly into the scraggle on his face, lines etched deep into his cheeks, and a look of sad resignation.

"Zade's here," he repeated. His throat was dry. The words croaked out. "He's over there, on the piano bench."

Lorrie didn't move, didn't change her expression, just continued her heavy breathing.

Doc stood, heaved and shoved the end of the bed to where she faced the piano bench without turning her head. The effort made his head ache, left him dizzy. He collapsed in his chair, rested his head on the edge of her mattress. His breath came in long, ragged wheezes. Lorrie's breathing grew quiet again. Doc lifted his head and stared with Lorrie at the empty piano bench.

Through the window, Doc noticed how the sunrise made a yellow border that outlined the mountain at the eastern edge of town. The oak tree had changed from a black silhouette to a dusky shadow. The yard was foggy, gray, like the darkness had stretched thin trying to reach from dusk to dawn, an extension of yesterday, the beginning of tomorrow.

"He was here," Doc said. "I saw him."

Lorrie stretched her skinny arm toward Doc. He leaned and reached between the bedrails. His gnarled fingertips brushed hers, like Adam's when he reached for God.

THE HEALER

Ike stood at his office window watching the sun, already well into its westward descent. He turned to his desk, moved his brief case to the floor from the chair where he had left it before daybreak, then looked around the room at the diplomas, certificates, and stacks of books. He flipped the pages of a medical journal, scanning the titles: deceptively precise descriptions of clinical research regarding the benefits of good blood pressure control, compulsive diabetes management, the proper treatment of a stroke.

Such precision once reassured him. The laws of nature were absolute, inflexible, brutally fair. The treatment of diabetes on the West Coast worked the same way it did on the East. The implications of a lump in the impoverished breast of a coal miner's wife were the same as if they were in the aristocratic breast of royalty. For every reaction there is an action, for every malady a treatment, for every cancer there was a scientifically derived cure waiting to be discovered.

He removed his clinic coat, starched and white when he started the day, now limp, wrinkled, used up. He sniffed at the sleeve, half expecting to smell the odor of decaying flesh or formaldehyde, smelling instead stale cigarette smoke and perfume, the blended aroma of the diverse clientele he served, old people reciting a litany of aches and pains, young people voicing fears and frustrations, poor people worrying about tomorrow, rich people unable to separate what they need from what they want.

Ike smiled bitterly, sank into his chair and swiv-eled to the desk, deciding as he moved that he would go back to the hospital before tackling the office work. He unwrapped a tuna salad sandwich that someone had left for him, sniffed it, started to drop it in the wastebasket, then reconsidered. He could not waste food, even when he wasn't hungry.

The stack of charts on his desk was already three days old before he added those for the patients he had seen today. Each of them needed a summary dictated. Some of them needed a review of the lab results he had ordered. Many of them would require a minor adjustment in medi-cine requiring a phone call. He enjoyed these conversations with his patients no matter how mundane. He rejoiced with them over good news, and he felt obligated to be the one to share the bad. Sometimes, he'd surprise an anxious patient to ask if they were tolerating their new medicine. If a patient died, he always called the spouse to offer his personal condolences. Recently, he'd had to delegate some of the more straight-forward calls to his very capable nurse.

He hadn't written notes in the hospital charts this morning. He had left that chore for his evening rounds, rationalizing that he would have something important to say if he waited. He started in the hospital early with the sickest of the sick, a menagerie of barely breathing bedrid-den people, caged behind chrome bed rails, some of them unable to speak for themselves, all dying from a unique but lethal mixture of bad genes, bad decisions, and bad luck. He was there before the phlebotomist drew their blood, before the consultants hauled them off for one procedure or another, so early that sometimes his patients wondered if they had dreamed Ike had laid his cold stethoscope on them in the dark and then whispered that he'd be back.

Ike knew that fear made the nights seem longer. He remembered how his asthma always seemed worse after dark, how he and his mother would sit and wait for Doc Haskins to knock, how the porch light formed a halo around him making the darkness behind him seem harmless, how his being there was as therapeutic as anything he carried in his tinkling black bag with its glass vials and syringes. Even when Ike knew his patients couldn't remember, even when they gave no sign that they recognized his presence, he always kept his whispered promise to return.

He was startled, but not surprised, to find Amy standing in his doorway. She worked part time, managed the phones in the afternoons, pulled the charts for the next day when the rest of the office staff was gone. Ike often exited an exam room or looked up from something he was reading to find her standing, waiting for his gaze to fall on her, or for him to somehow sense her presence. He wondered how long she had been watching him this time.

"Message for you, Doctor Corless," she said.

"Please, call me Ike," he said. Unlike the other doctors, he preferred that the office staff use his name. She probably didn't believe that he meant it, anyway. "And you don't need to wait for me to notice you when I'm obviously not busy," he continued, smiling. "Just knock or clear your throat or something. I might sit here looking out the window for hours."

"I know," she said. "But I forget."

Ike knew what she meant. Sometimes he felt like an intruder, too, like someone was waiting in the shadows to tell him that there had been a huge mistake, that he really hadn't graduated from medical school, hadn't excelled in an internal medicine residency, hadn't served as a medical officer in Vietnam, hadn't developed a busy practice while holding a faculty appointment at the University of Tennessee.

She handed him a pink sheet of paper torn from a message pad on which she had written in a neat, cursive font, "Call Preacher." She had drawn an upside-down question mark before and after it, then underlined each word several times with heavy pencil marks. Ike pictured her at the telephone politely trying to dissect the caller's identity, then the purpose and urgency of the call, making a new and heavier mark after each evasive answer.

Why couldn't Preacher just identify himself? Then again, why would he? Preacher was identification enough in Oak Grove. Just like Doc Haskins and Judge Goodman, Preacher's role in the community became who he was. Even Ike called him Preacher. He had never called him Dad.

"Is he still on the line?"

"No. I seen your office was empty when he called." She smiled and shrugged. "I thought you were still with a patient." She shifted her weight from one foot to the other. "Do you want me to call him back?."

"No," Ike said. "Thanks. I'll deal with it."

Ike and Preacher spoke to each other often, but they rarely talked. Their exchanges were never an opportunity to share, to chat, to enjoy the sound of each other's voice, to reminisce like a father and son. Ike called out of a sense of obligation. Preacher called as a reminder that Ike hadn't visited or to relay information about some catastrophe that God had meted on someone Ike sometimes faintly remembered. Preacher no longer interpreted these calamities as warning signs for Ike, but the subtext was still there.

Ike turned his chair to look out the window again. He watched the running lights on fishing boats, bobbing silent on the river. He often daydreamed about taking a Huck Finn trip, starting somewhere east of Knoxville on the French Broad or the Holston before they joined to form the Tennessee. He'd run at night, hide in the shallows during the day, avoid human contact, and follow the river to where the peaceful waters flow.

He had that feeling again when he dialed the number.

Preacher answered the phone on one ring. He didn't ask who was calling or say hello. "I need to talk to you," Preacher said.

Ike counted the files on his desk and remembered all the things he needed to do at the hospital.

"I need to see you in person. I need to talk to you, tonight," Preacher continued. There was genuine urgency in his voice, maybe fear, a sense of uncertainty that Ike recognized in his sickest patients.

The swirling silence between them broadened and deepened while Ike tried to organize an argument as to why he should put off a visit until the weekend. Before Ike could answer, Preacher used an evangelist's ploy, one exercised on the last night of a long series of revival services, used to force a decision from the most reluctant sinner, based on the uncertainty of the here and now, couching it against the certainty of the hereafter, of the wrath to come.

"Neither of us has the promise of tomorrow," he said.

Ike took the top down on his antique MGB, knowing that darkness did not assure a break in the heat. Knoxville had evolved to where it could block the sunlight but trap the heat, make a cloudless day seem gray and dirty, make a moonlit night seem muggy and hot. As he exited the parking garage and moved onto the street, Ike suppressed the urge to glance over his shoulder, imagined behind him a mass of people with shadowy, indistinct, faces with silent screaming mouths, with skeletal arms extended, and bony hands groping at him, trying to hold him back.

Oak Grove was less than a hundred miles from Knoxville, took less than two hours of driving even after maneuvering through the downtown traffic. The streets were still as bright as daytime from the light cast over them from the tall office buildings. When the glass and chrome towers faded out of his rearview mirror, the strip malls and restaurants lining Kingston Pike were just as bright. Only after he turned onto the open highway and headed toward the country did the path turn dark, marked only by the headlamps on his roadster, their reflection off road signs and billboards. Sporadic lights from modern homes cropped up in subdivided clumps where corn used to grow, and cattle once grazed.

The wind whipped at his hair and picked at his shirtsleeves. The forest crept in closer to the road. He smelled rich, mountain mulch and wet, rotting leaves. The cool air trapped in the evergreens poured over him. He pictured the river in the valley below, as invisible in the darkness as it was silent from his office window. He imagined that the road he traveled along the plateau mirrored its serpentine path.

Ike sped through the dark, recognizing, without seeing, tiny communities named Crab Orchard, Ozone Falls, and Mossy Cove and farms with barns whose sagging tin roofs served as billboards that read "Jesus Saves" on one side and "See Rock City" on the other. He passed churches made from remodeled white frame houses, labeled with hand-painted descriptive titles like "Glory Land Chapel" or "Church of the Mighty God." Some of them had little steeples perched over the former front porch as if to confirm the conversion from a house to a sanctuary.

The pastors of these churches, like Preacher, weren't shackled by denomination or doctrine, didn't answer to a deacon, a bishop, or a priest. During the day they were carpenters, coal miners, and farmers. At night they settled under dim lamps at wobbling kitchen tables and studied the onion-skin pages of their King James Version. They had no knowledge of the original Greek or Hebrew languages. They didn't own a commentary by a famous theologian, didn't need to know what someone else had written *about* the scripture. They listened and let the Bible speak for it-self. They parsed the message into sermons and preached, sometimes in their renovated houses, sometimes in converted carnival tents on the edge of town, and sometimes while standing on a street corner talking to people who would not meet their gaze.

Ike slowed and turned off the highway onto an even narrower road that led down the mountainside. Lightning flashed, revealing at once the mountains, the river and an opening in the forest on the valley floor that was Oak Grove, Tennessee. He could smell the rain. He considered racing the storm, gambling that he could drive the curvy road fast enough and that there would be time for him to put up the top without getting drenched when he reached Preacher's house. He thought better of it. Gravel crunched under the roadster's tires when he pulled onto the roadside and parked. He quickly unfolded the canvas roof, then snapped the metal grommets that held it in place.

The tires chirped on the pavement as he nosed the car back onto the road and accelerated. The luminous green gauges on his dashboard looked the way he imagined the cockpit of a WWII biplane flying at night. He worked through the gears, pushing the car, driving like he did when he was young and reckless. The guttural sound of the exhaust when he geared down marked his entry into one curve; the painful whine of the motor when he wound it tight coming out again marked the exit. White crucifixes made of painted wooden planks or Styrofoam, some of them draped with funeral wreaths, stood in the bend of the sharpest curves. The car seemed to descend almost as if Ike was not driving, as if it was moving under the direction of a higher power. The road fell behind him, twisting and turning, long and dark, like a bad memory.

The highway straightened at the foot of the mountain and led directly into town. Ike passed the clearing where Preacher Corless once held a tent revival every summer. Fireflies blinked in the clearing, reminding Ike of cigarettes hastily inhaled and doused by men finishing one last smoke before they went inside. He drove past the cemetery where a quarter-century earlier Ike had stood by his mother's casket, jaws clenched, teeth grinding, and Preacher stood by him, silently mouthing a prayer. It was threatening rain that day too.

After the funeral, Ike had retreated to his bedroom where Preacher found him packing clothes in a duffel bag.

"Where are you going?" Preacher asked.

Ike stuffed a shirt in the bag. "Away from here." He gestured, sweeping his arm around the room, toward the window, toward town. "Away from this."

"Away from here is a pretty big place," Preacher said.

"Good. So I can get far enough away that I don't have to hear you say, 'It's the Lord's will' every time something bad happens," he said. Ike crammed his shaving kit on top of the clothes and cinched the bag closed. "And when something good happens, it's a direct answer to your prayer."

Preacher reached toward Ike. "Let me explain…"

"Now you have your own prodigal son to preach about," Ike said, twisting away from Preacher's touch. He swung the bag to his shoulder. "Only, I don't want nothing you have, and I won't be coming back."

Ike turned off Main Street, followed a winding road past rusty mobile homes and dilapidated houses to the top of Tabernacle Hill, to the house where he was born. It was a simple place, well-kept compared to the neighbors. He paid a man to mow the lawn, to make repairs when needed. He paid a woman to cook and clean for Preacher, too. They no longer argued about it. It assuaged both of their consciences, Ike's checking on things and Preacher's letting him.

He parked the roadster and exited, stomped his penny loafers on the ground to start the circulation back in his feet, stretched, and savored the momentary discomfort in the muscles of his back. The misty scent of summer rain, so strong on the ride down the mountain, had changed to wet, heavy drops that drenched his shirt. He loosened his collar and was surprised to find his stethoscope still hanging around his neck.

The steep porch steps didn't look any more worn, didn't feel any ricketier than they did that hot August afternoon when Ike had stormed down them. He knocked on the doorframe. No one answered. He knocked again, harder. His knuckles stung. No answer. He yelled, "Hello?" His voice rose on the last syllable as if he were simultaneously greeting and asking a question. Still no answer.

He remembered the Bible story about the prodigal son. That father came to the edge of town to meet his wayward boy, gave him a ring, escorted him to the feast prepared in his honor. Preacher had called but now wouldn't answer... *Oh well... It was just a story.*

Ike opened the door and picked his way through familiar hallways. The feeling that he was traveling backward in time recurred, except that now he was not airborne and descending. Now he was softly, slowly being lowered into the claustrophobic confines of his childhood.

"Home sweet home," he whispered. The sound of his voice didn't reassure him.

He stopped at his old bedroom. The open door made the area seem larger. The faint fragrance of wintergreen liniment appeared from the dark corners of the room, as ominous as the cucumber smell that farmers claimed heralded the hidden presence of a copperhead. It transported him back to the nights he spent bolt upright in that bed wearing a poultice of Vicks Vapor Rub on his chest, holding his mother's hand while they waited for Doc

Haskins. He inhaled and held his breath for as long as he could.

Ike knew without looking that his baseball glove was on the top shelf of the closet. It would have been a fond memory in any other family, the way Ike's mother saved green stamps that the Quick Save Food Liner gave customers in return for buying groceries, the way she kept them in a shoe box until it was full, then sat at the kitchen table with a damp washcloth on a saucer beside her so she could moisten the stamps without licking them, the way she meticulously placed each stamp into the special booklet the store provided. It would have been a testimony to how poor people survive, the way she counted her booklets and studied the prize catalog, the way she agonized over whether to redeem an electric mixer, a toaster, or a set of plates with matching cups.

The summer Ike turned twelve, she traded three and a half booklets for a baseball glove. There was an autograph imprinted on the inside of the thumb, a name he didn't recognize as a boy and couldn't remember now. The pocket was shallow; the padding was so thin that, unless he snagged the ball precisely in the webbing, it offered no protection from anything more than the most dribbling line drive.

"Preacher," Eva said, while she cut Ike's birthday cake. "The boy wants to play in the Little League." Ike already had the uniform, a tee shirt with "Oak Grove First National Bank" written on the back in red, and a cap colored to match the letters.

Preacher ignored both of them, sat looking at his plate, holding his fork in his hand like a gavel.

Ike was encouraged that his mother seemed willing to push for this privilege, watched her sit down with her eyes level with Preacher's. She took a deep breath, started again. "He wants to play baseball...on a team. What harm can it do?"

Preacher looked away, into the distance, like he was studying a cloud on the horizon, one that looked innocent now, but might change abruptly into one that carried whipping winds, driving rain, thunder, and lightning.

"It's just a game; it's just little boys playing baseball," Eva said. "It's not the unpardonable sin." The knife with remnants of yellow cake and chocolate icing trembled in her hand.

Preacher's eyes moved toward Ike, as if to confirm what Eva had just told him, then they locked back on Eva for several seconds. Ike watched her gaze fall under the weight of his, saw her place the knife on the table with the resigned effect of a court-appointed lawyer shutting his briefcase after hearing his client's death sentence.

The cap was probably still in the closet too.

Ike moved farther down the hall to the room where his mother died, to the room where he knew he would find Preacher. Her memory hovered over him. He remembered how explosive her illness seemed, how her eyes and skin had turned yellow almost overnight, how her breath turned sickeningly sweet, how her belly swelled, stretching her bulky, loose-fitting Pentecostal clothes like something on the inside of her was fermenting.

Preacher went without sleep for the last three days of her life, carried her bedpan, coaxed her to eat, straightened her bed covers, placed cool compresses on her forehead. Ike sat on the other side of her bed, held her hand, kissed her cheek, did all the unnecessary, tender touching, all the unimportant things that let her know that she was not alone, and that he was already lonely.

Preacher had lost a lot of weight since Ike's last visit. His facial bones, visible under the thin layer of skin drawn tight over them, framed eyes that still glowed with religious fervor. His hair was white and wispy instead of the lush coal-black growth that Ike had inherited from him. A stack of pillows held him upright. An over-the-bed table held his black leather Bible, the same one he studied when Ike was a boy. Jesus looked down at the bed from a framed picture hanging on the wall, compassionate and concerned. Preacher was so pale that Ike could trace the small, lacy blood vessels visible in his eyelids even in the dim yellow light.

"How are you, Preacher?" he asked. He could think of nothing better, nothing more neutral to say.

"Spiritually, I'm fine, son, but the flesh is weak." His husky voice seemed to echo from the cadaverous face. His voice sounded stronger than it did on the phone. Ike moved closer to the bed, observed Preacher clinically while he talked. "I'm glad you called me back, Isaac." He paused, breathing in short, shallow respirations between pursed lips. The effort caused beads of perspiration to form on his forehead. He mopped at his face with a bandana like the one he used when he preached revivals. That familiar motion evoked a memory so strong that Ike wondered if the raindrops beating on the roof were real or imagined.

"How long has that been happening?"

"I've been having sweats for five or six weeks. I've only been short-winded for a couple of days." Preacher stopped talking to breathe for a few seconds. "I ain't been able to get out of bed today." He closed his eyes. "I'm glad you came home, son," he said. "I prayed that you would."

Ike studied Preacher, while he listened to the rain pecking against the windows, somehow knowing that the wind would soon be lashing the trees outside. He felt a twinge of pity for this old man who still believed he could change the natural course of events by his prayers.

"Let me take a look at you," Ike said.

Preacher withdrew into the pillows. "I didn't call you here to doctor on me, son. Doc Haskins came out today and give me a shot. I'm better. You don't need to do nothing medical. Sit down. Just hear me out."

Ike had never examined Preacher, had never wanted to. It didn't seem natural, somehow, to touch someone who had spent a lifetime keeping his distance, staying just out of reach. He wanted to let it go this time, but he couldn't. "I promise, I won't do anything that embarrasses us," he said, hoping to hide his own discomfort under a clinical mask. "At least let me listen to your heart and lungs."

Without waiting for an answer, he moved to the bedside. He noted the dry, cracked lips, the plaque coating Preacher's tongue. Even feeling through his thick flannel pajama top, Ike found a grapelike cluster of rubbery lymph glands in each skeletal armpit. He lifted the shirt in the back, placed his stethoscope on Preacher's chest, listened to his lungs ripping and tearing like Velcro with every breath. Ike helped him recline, amazed at how small Preacher seemed compared to the evangelist who still towered in his memories. He leaned over to open Preacher's shirt just enough to place the stethoscope over his heart.

Preacher put his hand on Ike's. "Please. Let me talk first." As he pushed Ike's hand, the stethoscope bell hung on the shirt, pulling the top of it open, uncovering a scar that started at the lower part of Preacher's neck and disappeared down his chest, under the pajama top. Ike jerked away from Preacher's feeble grip. He opened the shirt, pulled roughly at each button, exposed Preacher's chest. He ran his finger the length of the scar. Through the skin, Ike could feel the wires a surgeon had placed to hold Preacher's breastbone together after heart surgery.

Ike walked to the window putting as much distance between himself and Preacher as the room allowed. He clenched his teeth until his jaws ached.

"I guess I didn't realize that the Great Physician was a heart surgeon," Ike said.

"Do not blaspheme in this house," Preacher said. When Ike didn't answer, he continued, "This happened when you were away, in the Army…if you care to hear about it."

Ike raised the windowpane to let the air circulate. He could see the trees swaying back and forth, their movements choreographed by the storm. Bits of hymns, fragments of Bible verses gusted into his mind. Across town, beyond the railroad tracks, he imagined a revival tent glowing golden through the darkness. The last church service that Ike had attended, other than his mother's funeral, played again in his mind like a movie.

Hot July raindrops beat on the canvas roof as Preacher Corless walked slowly to the makeshift pulpit. His shoulders sagged under the burden of his message. He surveyed the audience from under thick, black eyebrows and swiped his forehead with a large handkerchief.

Eva Corless sat in the front row, her eyes closed. A strand of hair trailed down her back to the waist. A puff of wind irreverently billowed her skirt. Another gust caused a rush of raindrops to pound on the canvas rooftop, sprayed the people sitting near the open sides of the tent. Cicadas buzzed in the darkness. Preacher searched each member of the congregation separately and together. He took off his coat and tossed it on a chair behind him. He removed his necktie, rolled his sleeves up around his elbows, like he was getting ready to wrestle or dig a ditch. He talked earnestly, in a deep monotone, punctuated occasionally with a groan. He developed a spellbinding cadence to his oration, which became more prominent as he lost himself in the sermon. He drenched his shirt with sweat, raked his hair backward, away from his eyes, with whichever hand did not hold his Bible. He preached until his breath came in heavy, rapid gasps, until he was too tired to continue.

Preacher dried his face with his handkerchief while the congregation moved forward, leaving Ike on the back bench, exposed and alone. Eva sat with her hands folded in her lap, her eyes closed like she was in a trance. Everyone strained to reach her, to place a hand on some part of her. Preacher dabbed a drop of olive oil on her forehead with his index finger, then covered the spot with the palm of his hand while he prayed.

"Lord, we know that healing is a spiritual gift," he said. "Some people never find it. Some people don't look. But the gift is there. We just have to have the faith to claim it." He paused; even the cicadas were silent, as if in deference to Preacher's prayer. "So, I come asking you to heal my wife. I've come to You, Lord, the Great Physician. Reward us, right now, I pray. Let her be an example of Your power and glory."

The tender gesture, the simple prayer, the whole image was unlike anything Ike had ever witnessed between Preacher and Eva. His heart pounded. His pulse raced. For an instant, he let himself believe he was feeling the pulsating rhythm of hope.

The service closed with the congregation singing an invitation hymn, one written in the 1800s describing the plight of a sinner who had considered but declined the offer of eternal life. Ike walked out of the tent, across the muddy parking lot, toward the lights of town. "Almost persuaded, now to receive," they sang. He broke into a run. "Almost persuaded, now to believe..." floated behind him in the humid night air.

Preacher's voice interrupted Ike's reverie. "I started having angina right after your momma died. Doc Haskins treated me with medicine for a long time, then the attacks came back and was even waking me at night. I prayed for healing. It seemed like my prayers just hit the ceiling and bounced back down on me. I was desperate, I reckon. Maybe I didn't wait on the Lord's will." He breathed heavily for a moment, then opened his eyes, suddenly, as if it surprised him that Ike had stayed. "Doc Haskins got me an appointment with a heart doctor in Nashville. You was in the Army. I made him promise not to let you know unless something happened to me."

Ike paced back and forth the length of the bedroom, taking deep breaths and letting them out slowly, like he had learned to do as a boy. He mopped his forehead with his sleeve. Each heartbeat seemed to pound blood deeper and deeper into his brain.

"What about Mom?" Ike asked, each word rasping in his throat like sandpaper on wood. "What's the difference in you and her?"

"Her faith was stronger than mine. That's what." Preacher rested his head back on his pillows, exhausted. "I tried to get her to see Doc Haskins. Ask him, if you don't believe me. He came out here more than once and talked to her." Preacher rested again.

"She might be alive…"

"Maybe so. Medicine could of controlled things for a while. She knew that." He paused to breathe, closed his eyes. "That ain't the same as healing. My surgery was a miracle, but I wasn't healed. My chest pains went away, but I still had heart problems." He rested, then continued in a whisper, "Your mom got something better. God took her physical body and gave her a spiritual one, perfect in every way." Preacher's eyes flashed again, and his voice became almost strident. "I couldn't've dealt with her dying the way she did if I didn't have that to hold on to."

Ike didn't answer.

Preacher coughed and winced, holding his ribs. He tried to fluff his pillows so he could sit upright.

Ike moved helplessly back to the window. The sun rising in the east caused the earth to glow again. Preacher continued talking, barely penetrating Ike's trance, his present words confluent with the sermon Ike remembered from years ago.

"That's the difference in earthly physicians and the Great Physician. All things work together for good with the Great Physician. They's a trade-off when you earthly doctors get involved." He closed his eyes again and breathed quietly for a while.

Ike kept looking out the window.

"I still believe He can heal," Preacher said. His voice faded into a husky whisper.

The pattering raindrops on the rooftop settled into a steady rhythm. Ike turned away from the window, watched his father, head back on the pillows, barely breathing. He pulled a chair close to the bed, placed his hand on Preacher's brow, felt the oily moisture cling to his fingertips. Preacher roused, tried to focus his black eyes on Ike like he had on congregations in years past. His eyelids were too heavy. They fluttered shut. Ike searched under the quilt for Preacher's wrist, felt his thready pulse. He didn't resist when his dad's hand moved to hold his. They sat that way for a long time. It surprised Ike how naturally it happened, how comforted he felt, how he was almost persuaded to believe.

Heart Sounds

After the night Preacher and I reconciled, he rallied a little, or at least seemed to be dying slower. I stayed over a couple of days to arrange twenty-four hour caregivers so I could go back to work, but after the second morning that I found him in the hallway floor halfway from his bed to the bathroom, I drove back to Knoxville, met with my partners and told them I needed an extended leave of absence. They were sympathetic, but not happy. They would have to divide my practice, and I couldn't tell them for how long. I felt guilty, but there was no alternative.

My car was parked outside, packed with as much as I could cram in the trunk, tie onto the luggage rack and pile into the passenger seat. I was exhausted by the time I completed my round trip from Oak Grove to Knoxville and back. I stopped on the edge of town, at the Peggy Ann, to fuel up and eat before settling in at Preacher's house.

Business was booming at the truck stop. Two men stood on ladders looking at the motor of a large tractor-trailer with its cab tilted forward. Metal clanged on metal from inside the garage. Every breath I took came loaded with the taste of diesel fuel.

"Food pretty good in the restaurant?" I asked as the attendant gave me change.

He studied my wrinkled khaki pants, penny loafers and unbuttoned button-down collar. "If you like breakfast," he said.

I pulled away from the pumps, parked my MGB closer to the restaurant and walked inside. Red booths lined the walls. Thick-waisted truckers wearing greasy baseball caps hunkered over huge plates of steaming scrambled eggs, flakey white biscuits and sausage-gravy. They held their forks like garden tools then dipped their head down to meet the load halfway.

I moved to a corner booth. The one-page menu had a sketch of an 18-wheeler in the background with a typewritten list of choices. A sign over the cash register read, "Breakfast served 24 hours."

A cup of coffee with steam curling off the rim appeared in front of me. Two small plastic containers of cream rolled across the table and landed by the cup. The waitress hitched her hip and took an order pad from the rear pocket of her jeans.

"My name is Jamie," she said. "I'll be your server." The lilting line sounded more appropriate to one of the upscale restaurants near the university where co-eds with trust funds worked. I looked up, straight into sky blue eyes that mocked me.

I squirmed in my seat, trying hard to think of something clever to say. The plastic squeaked under my trousers. Blood rushed to my face.

Jamie laughed. "Lordy Ike…you ain't changed a bit."

Her face rearranged from happy to sad while she wiped an imaginary wet spot on my table. She turned to me. Her lips actually moved, but nothing came out, like she had thought better of it after the command left her brain but before the words left her mouth.

She moved to another table, without saying anything.

We had exchanged letters after I went to college. Her sentences with "ain't" and "I seen" announced the pregnancies and marriages of our Oak Grove classmates. It was a stark contrast to my new friends who carefully pronounced the "ing" on the end of their words and who were equally concerned with world hunger and getting their own apartments.

I studied her while she worked. She looked as pretty as she did in her senior picture in the Oak Grove Miners Yearbook, Class of 1965.

"Can I getcha anything else, love?" she asked a bald-headed man with three days of stubble on his face.

He said something that I couldn't hear.

She laughed and put her hand lightly on his arm. A tattoo of a snake circled his wrist, forearm and shoulder. Its angry eyes and flickering tongue threatened me from the broad part of his shoulder exposed by a plaid button-down shirt with the sleeves ripped off. She whispered something back, then tore the order ticket off her tablet and slapped it next to his plate.

"Bye, Hon," she said. "See you on the flip-flop."

The trucker winked and left a tip that was twice the cost of his meal.

She turned back to me. "You look like you just lost your puppy," she said. "What'sa matter?"

Behind her, the trucker stood tucking his shirttail into jeans that barely covered his butt.

"Not having that which having makes one happy," I said.

"Well, hey-lo, Mr. Shakespeare," she said. "You always was Mrs. Haskins' favorite."

I wanted to take her in my arms and slow dance like we did at the senior prom while the jukebox played Carole King singing "Will You Still Love Me Tomorrow?" I wanted to waltz down the aisle past the grazing truckers, through the diesel fumes in the parking lot, out to the evergreens where the fall foliage rustled on the ground, and backward through time to when she was mine.

She punched me softly on my shoulder. "You gonna order or what?"

Her wedding band burned through my starched cotton shirt like a branding iron.

Preacher didn't like it, but I examined him every day, just like I did my hospital patients. Each morning, his heart sounded weaker and more apathetic. His lungs sounded like Velcro ripping and tearing with each breath.

The jagged scar on his chest from his heart surgery made us both uneasy. I'd found the scar the first time I had examined him, before he'd had a chance to explain. Doc Haskins had convinced him to have bypass surgery when he developed chest pain from heart blockages while we were estranged.

I forgave him. I had to work at it. I still do. I can't get past how my mom died with metastatic cancer waiting for divine intervention twenty-five years ago with what I believed until very recently was Preacher's tacit approval.

He lived his last days propped bolt upright on his pillows. Every breath was a work of faith. The house reeked of Vicks liniment from a poultice he insisted I make and hang on his chest like my mother did for me when I had croup. It didn't work for me. I don't think it worked for Preacher. It gave us both the sense that something was being done.

His wet breathing rattled in a pattern I recognized, a long pause, sometimes thirty seconds or more, then slow and deep, then fast, then faster, followed by another long pause. I tried to hold my breath each time his breathing stopped. My mind tried to force me to breathe long before his coaxed him to take another deep breath and resume his cycle. Mom's breathing just kept getting shallower and shallower. When she stopped, people in the room kept whispering to each other and dabbing at their eyes with Kleenex for five minutes before anyone noticed she was gone.

Preacher's fear of suffocation escalated as he declined. Sundown panic attacks and nocturnal delirium became so predictable that Doc Haskins came by every evening to give him an injection and save a middle of the night visit.

"Good day or bad?" Doc asked me as he dropped his medical bag on the floor and leaned over to feel for Preacher's pulse.

"He's sleeping a lot during the day," I said.

I was trying to explain why Preacher had been awake so much at night. Doc thought I was asking him to do something.

He put his antique stethoscope on Preacher's chest and kept talking. "I slept all day...the birds do thus...The unhappy days I choose to sleep," he said. As he turned back to me, the heavy bell of his stethoscope floated in an arc from its tether on his neck. It settled harmlessly on his belly. "Or something like that." Doc was not a man who read poetry, but his wife had been my high school English teacher and he quoted her often.

He sat down with his back straight, one hand on each knee, his black doctor bag on the floor beside him.

"Good day or bad, Preacher?" he asked.

"The flesh is weak," Preacher answered.

"The Spirit is strong," Doc said, just the way Preacher coached him.

Jesus looked down at the two of them with a satisfied smile from the picture over the head of Preacher's bed.

The Oak Grove Medical Clinic was a renovated house that inhabited some family's memory as a home during the 50s. The front yard was a gravel parking lot. There was an unpainted wooden ramp that led to the porch from the left and wooden steps on the right. It wasn't even ten a.m., but the waiting room was packed with people sitting around the walls in straight back chairs looking at people who were looking at them from chairs lining the middle of the room. Doc didn't set appointments. He just worked until people quit signing the clipboard hanging at the check-in window.

"Sign the list," she said, when I asked the receptionist if I could speak to Doc Haskins.

"I'm a doctor," I said. "I need to speak to him."

She unsheathed a sharp edge to her voice. "Then sign in," she said, "and have a seat."

We were glaring at each other when the door from the clinical area opened. Doc worked faster than his nurse, so he often called his patients back himself.

"Deacon?" he said to the entire room at the same time he saw me.

A short scrawny man wearing bib overalls stood.

"I came by to ask you a favor," I said. "If you have time." I looked around the room and felt silly. Deacon jockeyed into position next to Doc, careful not to lose his place to me. The receptionist snorted behind me.

"You'll need to wait a little bit," he said to me, louder than necessary. "I've gotta give the deacon his gonorrhea shot."

Doc Haskins' laughter followed the receptionist and me to his office.

"He's an awful busy man," I said, trying not to gloat. "But he sure seems to enjoy it."

She pointed to a chair, turned her chin up and walked out.

Doc entered thirty minutes later, swiping at his hands with a paper towel. I sensed he had forgotten about me because I'd heard him call back three or four other people, and his nurse called at least two more. He even played the gonorrhea joke again on somebody.

"Good morning," he said.

The speech I had rehearsed about my appreciation for the way he treated my dad, my desire to contribute to a real community with real needs, my yearning to relieve human suffering…just evaporated.

"I want to come home," I said.

Doc studied me as if I had just described a pain for which there was no anatomic explanation.

"Lorrie used to say that home is the place that when you go there, they have to take you back," he said without smiling. I recognized it as another line from Robert Frost, but Doc only knew what Mrs. Haskins taught him.

Doc studied his fingers like he was rehearsing the names of the bones. His eyes had an otherworld gaze.

"You married?"

My divorce wasn't final, so yes was technically the truth.

"It's not easy, being a small-town doctor and a family man."

I nodded, careful to say enough but not too much.

"Lorrie liked the poem about the fork in the road…" Doc left long pauses between his sentences, like he was inviting me to interrupt. There's a line where the poet tells himself he can come back and take the other path even though he knows he probably won't."

I thought of Jamie.

"Don't bet on it," he said, as if he'd read my mind.

Doc continued to study me, like he was trying to figure out why anyone who got away from Oak Grove would want to come back. He turned to his bookshelf. It sagged under the burden of textbooks and journals he had stacked, many unwrapped, still in their plastic mailing slips. He slipped a 33-rpm vinyl record out of its faded jacket and put it on an old phonograph next to his desk.

"I'd been here a couple of years before I decided I wanted to be a heart specialist," he said.

He set the needle arm on the record.

"I ordered this recording of heart sounds so I could learn the pathologic murmurs."

There was a rhythmic scratching sound before the needle seated in the groove, then the room was full of lubs and dubs and whooshes interspersed with a professorial voice identifying the distinctive features of mitral stenosis or aortic insufficiency.

Doc gestured toward the now standing room only waiting area. "I couldn't leave."

Silence took root between us. I let it grow as I remembered how Mrs. Haskins took the summers and toured foreign countries while Doc stayed home and worked. Her Kodachrome slide show in school assembly every fall, with pictures of her on the back of an elephant or standing next to a pyramid or bartering in a third world marketplace, documented the roads she had traveled. Doc sat in the back of the auditorium and watched with the rest of us.

The crescendo and decrescendo rush of a recorded heart murmur I didn't recognize swirled in the silence between us. "I've listened to everybody's heart in this valley," he said. "Except mine."

I parked in a clump of trees about a half mile from Jamie's little white house on Airport Road while I waited for the sun to drop a little further. Earlier, I had seen her crossing the parking lot at the IGA grocery as I was placing my bags in the passenger seat of my car. Her long legs, her honey brown hair, her faded jeans, and her breezy walk almost made me fail to notice the man with her. He was tall, thin, roughhewn, dressed in work boots, jeans and a shirt with a white patch over his left pocket with the name Billy Sawyer stitched in a cursive font. They loaded their groceries into an old, but well-kept Ford F-150 pickup parked next to my MG.

While Billy secured their packages, Jamie came around to get in the passenger seat. We were so close I could have put my arms around her.

"Hi Jamie," I said.

She looked at me, nodded and smiled but didn't say anything as she shut the door.

"How'd he know your name?" Billy said. I could hear him clearly over the low powerful rumble of the truck engine.

"He's just someone I used to know," she said.

I drove back to the clinic, located Jamie's medical record and jotted down her address on the back of an envelope. I knew the place. I'd driven past it while making house calls for Doc Haskins. I sat with her chart in my lap flipping through her life recorded in Doc's handwritten scrawl, from birth, to marriage, to childbirth, to routine encounters for one thing or another.

I got up and found Billy's record. I don't know what I hoped to find, maybe that he had only a few months to live, or that Doc Haskins had actually treated him for a venereal disease, something to give me an excuse to make a play for Jamie. There was nothing there but a physical exam for a life insurance policy he'd bought ten years earlier.

I left my car and walked through the woods, then settled in the shadows directly across the road from Jamie's front porch. Lights punched holes in the darkness through one window after another. A television flickered in the front room.

The front door opened, and Jamie sat down on the front porch steps with a blanket draped around her shoulders. Billie followed and sat down beside her. They snuggled under the blanket. I squatted there in the darkness with my legs aching, afraid to move. I was so close I could hear the hum and mumble of their voices whispering back and forth.

After a while, two boys, twelve or thirteen years old, came outside wearing pajamas. They giggled and talked, then hugged Jamie, and then Billie.

"Git in the bed," Billy said. "Tomorrow's a school day."

The boys laughed and ran back inside the house. The screen door slammed behind them.

I imagined how it would feel to be under that blanket with Jamie, whispering whatever people do when they live for each other. I tried to picture how the boys would look if they were mine, how it would feel to have their unbridled love and to return it without conditions.

Jamie and Billy sat for a while longer. When they stood, their two shadows merged, then separated as they turned inside. One by one, the window lights disappeared.

I shivered. October in the mountains can be cool, especially when you've sat without moving for two hours. I stood, stretched and stomped the feeling back into my feet. I stumbled through the woods barely able to see the path that I'd followed earlier despite a clear and moonlit night. I found my car with the groceries still riding in the passenger seat, coasted it onto the road, popped the clutch, started the engine and headed home, knowing that the thing which having would have made me happy was just someone I used to know.

I couldn't decide whether Jamie had influenced my decision to come home more than I realized or my fear of someday meeting her as a patient had scared me away. Six months had vanished, and I still hadn't told Doc Haskins that I'd decided to see if I could rejoin my old practice in Knoxville.

When I opened the door to the exam room and saw her profile outlined by the sterile fluorescent light, I was just as stunned as when we met in the Peggy Ann. Her dress hung loose enough to hide the details. Her face was pale. She had dark circles under her eyes. She had wound her hair into a knot of some sort, low on the back of her neck.

I leaned slightly to steady myself on the corner of the exam table. I nodded to Billy, seated on a chair in the corner, elbows on his knees, hands fidgeting with his cap.

"Are you OK?" she asked.

I took another deep breath. "Yes."

She smiled. "You're supposed to ask me that."

There was not enough room in my chest to talk and breathe at the same time. "I didn't expect you," I said. I took another breath. "You surprised me."

Her gaze drifted downward. "Billy made me come," she said.

My face burned again. How much had she told him? Had she told him anything?

"She's bleeding," Billy said, from behind me.

Jamie looked past me toward the window, as if hearing what Billy said was worse than just knowing it.

"Your periods?" I blurted.

She paused while I finished congratulating myself on having solved her problem before I had heard all of it.

"That too." She took a long breath. "I saw Doc Haskins last month because I didn't feel good. I was tired all the time. He told me my blood was low and gave me a vitamin."

I paged slowly through her chart. Doc had diagnosed iron deficiency and placed her on supplements without ordering any lab.

"Now I'm having nose bleeds, and I bruise for no reason. It's been getting worse. I'm to the point I can hardly drag myself around. I ain't been able to work in two weeks."

I gave Jamie time to change into a gown while I tried to locate someone to stand in the room with me while I examined her.

"No one's accused me of anything in over 50 years," Doc said, the first time I mentioned I wasn't comfortable examining women without a chaperone. "They either trust you or they don't."

Doc Haskins's nurse came back in with me and stood quietly by the door.

"You want me to leave?" Billy asked.

"Jamie might be more comfortable with you here," I said.

Billy settled back again and studied his hat.

Jamie sat at the end of the table with her back straight, her bare feet kicking back and forth slightly.

I felt disorganized, disjointed, as apprehensive and amateurish as a first-year med student doing his first exam on a live patient. I touched her face, turned it straight toward me and avoided her eyes while I examined her pale conjunctiva.

"Let me look in your mouth," I said.

Dried blood outlined her lower teeth. A slight pressure on her gums caused them to ooze a little. It embarrassed her.

I traced down her neck, over her shoulders, under her arms, feeling for lymph glands. I studied her hands, the perfect symmetry of the fingertips, the translucent skin. I remembered their soft, electric touch. I moved the gown, traced down her thighs covered with old and new bruises the size of silver dollars, down to her shins covered with little purple dots no larger than a pin head, to her feet, where I caressed a scar on the instep of the right one where she cut it on a sharp rock while we waded a stream on the backside of Marion Ridge during our last year of high school.

She pulled her foot away.

I blushed.

Billy picked at a string on his cap.

I had her lie back on the table. My eyes drifted downward toward the soft bulge of her breasts under the skimpy gown. She had her eyes closed, fingers intertwined across her belly like it was Sunday afternoon and we were lying on a blanket in the grass by the river. She let me guide her hands to her sides, out of the way, so I could palpate her stomach. When I placed my stethoscope on her chest, she opened her eyes and searched mine while I listened to her heart.

My hematology colleagues in Knoxville assured me that Doc Haskins delayed her treatment but didn't change her menu of options by misdiagnosing Jamie's leukemia as iron poor blood. That's a kind way of saying her prognosis is so bad that it's merciful to live for a while in ignorance.

I struggled with the same anger about Doc's judgment as I did when I thought Preacher was complicit in my mother's decision to wait for divine intervention as her treatment plan.

When I confronted him, he removed his wire rim glasses. The wrinkles in his face rearranged themselves into a profound caricature of sadness. He melted into his chair, covered his face with his hands. "I was there when she was born. I delivered her boys. I've known her all her life." Doc looked up at me without moving anything but his eyes. "How can this be?" he whispered. "How did I not see this?"

I imagined him back when he was thinking of leaving to become a heart specialist, his big broad shoulders bent over a farmer's naked chest, his brow furrowed, listening to his memory of the sounds on the heart murmur album, comparing them to the live ones in his stethoscope. I envisioned all the babies he'd delivered, the cumulative number of cuts, scrapes and breaks he'd treated as they grew up and had children of their own, the wealth of good will he'd accrued, the gratification of having practiced in his hometown, all negated by the devastation of one error in judgment. These were his people, the reasons he once considered leaving. They were also the reasons he decided not to go.

Neither of us could speak. I turned to his bookcase and located the record. The phonograph needle made its rhythmic scratching sound while the stentorian voice of a long dead professor introduced "a holosystolic murmur that radiates from the apex of the heart to the axilla."

I don't know why, but I leaned over Doc and placed my stethoscope on his chest. He jerked, the way Preacher did the first time I listened to him, but he didn't resist. His eyes searched mine, like Jamie's did when I examined her. I held my breath. While the harsh murmurs from the phonograph blended with the rhythm of his tired heart, I struggled to listen to my own.

THE LONG WAY HOME

Imogene stood at the kitchen door looking into the garage at her husband's ghost behind the steering wheel of his old Chevrolet. He was a happy man when alive, and he loved to drive. He'd put one hand on the steering wheel, prop his other on the window edge, and push his hat back as if he hadn't a care in the world. Sometimes, she'd send him to the grocery to get a carton of milk, and he'd return three hours later without the milk or any memory of where he'd been.

"I took the long way home," he'd say, as if that said it all.

He looked so serious now, didn't wave, didn't smile, didn't acknowledge her. He kept both hands on the wheel and his eyes fixed straight ahead, like there was a hard road to drive and not much time to drive it.

The first time, he had frightened her. She slammed the door shut, ran to his closet, and sifted through his shirts, pants, and coats, still hanging as they did when he was alive. She found his hat on the top shelf, the same hat she remembered him wearing in the car. She held it, examined it inside and out, sniffed the year-old sweat stains, and found two gray hairs still lodged in the lining. She found his pipe, still pungent with the stale odor of burnt Sir Walter Raleigh tobacco.

"I knew it," she said. "I'm seeing things." She said it out loud, like exposing her thoughts to oxygen revealed her mind's treachery, like saying it so she could hear it provided her with another witness. She placed the pipe and the hat on the table near her chair where she could touch them and smell them whenever she wanted.

Imogene's son Tom encouraged her to drive the car after the funeral. She couldn't do it.

"It feels like Jesus is sitting in the passenger seat," she said. "The only place it'll take me is to the church and the cemetery."

For the year since Carl died, except when Tom took it for a drive, the car stayed in the garage, where Imogene could see it and touch it if she wanted. It was only during the past few weeks that his image appeared behind the wheel with anything that caused a memory of him.

The January wind blew under the garage door strong enough to lift the hem of her dress. Cold air touched the skin above her knees where she had her stockings knotted. The sensation startled her. She jerked her hands down to smooth her dress. Her vision blurred. She yielded to a swirling awareness of falling, flailing, the anticipation of an impact certain to break bones followed by a feeling like she was waking from a nightmare with no memory of the dream.

There were multiple bruises but no fractures. She was only in the hospital a few days. Doctor Corless, who had graduated high school with Imogene's son Tom and his wife Lacy, wanted to send her to Shannondale.

"If your blood sugar gets too high again," he warned, "you might not be so lucky. It would only be a temporary thing. You can go home when you get a little stronger."

Even though he said "when," she knew he really meant "if." Doc Haskins had said the same thing to Carl, after his stroke.

"Reckon me and Lacy could take care of her at home for a while?" Tom asked.

Imogene tried to imagine Tom wearing shiny penny loafers, khaki pants and a shirt with a button-down collar. She wondered if he felt self-conscious with his calloused hands and his job servicing cars at the Chevrolet dealership in Knoxville.

"You live twenty miles away," Doctor Corless said. "You both work. That's a lot of driving."

"Me and Lacy's talked about it. We could move in for a while, if we need to. I think we'd like to try, just till we see how it goes."

I'll be waiting on them hand and foot in two days.

"What about letting me get her some visiting nurses, then?" Doctor Corless answered.

Home nurses? Strangers traipsing through the house will be worse than Tom and Lacy being there, Imogene thought.

"I'm OK now," she said. "My eyes ain't blurry anymore. I was just eating wrong and my blood sugar went up. I don't need nurses. Tom and Lacy can help me."

She looked at her feet, covered in a pair of thick white athletic socks, the only thing that would keep her toes warm. *Why does keeping control of my sugar mean losing control of everything else?*

Tom wheeled Carl's old Chevy into the hospital parking area. Lacy was leaning on his shoulder, still wearing her nursing aide uniform with the orange University Hospital logo on the sleeve. Tom wore a baseball cap riding on the back of his head with his thick brown hair sticking out around the edges.

The attendant helped Imogene from the wheelchair. Her pink flannel gown hung below her long winter coat. Her heavy socks stretched the fluffy pink house shoes made to match her gown. Tom loaded her suitcase into the trunk, then grinned at her.

"You want to go for a little drive?" he asked.

"Take the long way home," she said. She almost called him Carl.

Tom cradled Imogene's frail little hand in his, pricked her finger and squeezed out a drop of blood. He had organized her diabetes care just as if he was going down the maintenance checklist on a luxury car.

"That hurt?" he asked. He didn't wait for an answer, but squinted at the glucose meter, then recorded her sugar level on a homemade flow sheet.

"It don't feel good," she said. "I think you're doing it too much. My fingers are so sore and my arms ache."

Tom frowned and nodded as if he wasn't pleased with where the last number landed on his graph.

"I feel fine," she said. "So my blood sugars are fine."

Lacy bought a microwave and filled the refrigerator with frozen dinners. "We need to follow a strict diabetic diet," she said, like the food Imogene cooked for sixty years was slowly poisoning her. "We want 'heart healthy' meals from now on."

"I don't eat thawed-out food," Imogene said. "That's how people get ptomaine poisoning." She pressed her lips together in a thin line, folded her arms across her chest. *Let them look that up,* she thought. *I know a few medical things, too.*

"It's just to make it easier for you," Tom said. "We're just trying to do things so you can stay by yourself. We thought that's what you wanted."

"I ain't helpless," Imogene said.

"Is Shannondale as bad as it used to be?" she asked after Doctor Corless perched on his stainless-steel stool, Imogene's clinic record on his lap. She almost called him Ike but thought better of it.

He laughed. "I don't know how bad it used to be. Have you changed your mind about being at home?"

"No. But me being home is complicating things. Tom and Lacy are trying to work in Knoxville and take care of me here in Oak Grove. It's hard on them. I ain't used to being a burden."

"Maybe if you'd let me get you some help, visiting nurses, some equipment, it might take the pressure off Tom and Lacy."

"Equipment?" She pictured an iron lung or a motorized wheelchair.

"Like a hospital bed, shower stool, commode extender."

"Oh." She blushed. Commode was a word she was too embarrassed to say louder than a whisper, even when she had to call a plumber. She wondered how Doctor Corless knew that she struggled every time she went to the bathroom, how she strained to stand up from her toilet seat, how she had envisioned herself being trapped, sitting on that hard plastic oversized horseshoe for hours, her bloomers around her ankles, waiting for Tom or Lacy or the Oak Grove volunteer fire department to break the door down and rescue her.

"Home nurses could check your blood sugar, too," he continued.

That's it, she thought. That's why Tom didn't argue about waiting outside. They had already talked.

Imogene bristled. "I don't need anyone to check my blood sugar for me. I can tell if it's up or down by the way I feel."

Dr. Corless smiled. "What is it now?"

She hesitated, then said, "What is *what* now?"

"Your blood sugar. Is it up or down, right now?"

"I feel just fine," she said.

"So it's good?" Doc Corless reached over, took her middle finger, pricked it, and ran the test strip right there in the exam room. The level was more than twice normal. "See? You can't tell what your blood sugar is by the way you feel. You need to let someone help you with it. Otherwise, you'll be back in the hospital, then you probably will wind up in Shannondale, or worse."

Imogene wilted. *A person ought to be able to know how they feel,* she thought. *A person shouldn't have to wonder, shouldn't feel all right, but not be all right.* She didn't argue when Doctor Corless brought Tom back to update him personally. She gathered her things and limped away while they talked, then stopped, leaned on her walker and stared out the window. Tom had parked the Chevy close to the building in a handicapped parking slot. Carl's image appeared behind the wheel. She looked back over her shoulder to where Tom and Ike were talking and laughing as if they were still in high school. When she looked back, Carl was gone. She wondered if her blood sugar being up would make her see things that weren't really there.

"The dining room is the only room big enough for a hospital bed," Tom said.

"And it has a view out on the front yard, plus it's convenient to the kitchen," Lacy said. "She won't have to walk so far to get her meals."

Imogene pretended she didn't hear them since they were talking as if she wasn't there. Tom had loaded her antique table and chairs onto his truck to make room for a hospital bed. He moved her reclining rocker from the back bedroom to the window in the converted dining room, and the television she never watched where she could see it anytime. He placed her electric space heater where it aimed directly at the spot where she would rest her feet.

"You be careful with that heater," Lacy said to him. "Diabetics have numb feet, and she could burn herself without knowing it."

So. I'm not even a person anymore. I'm a type of person, probably one with dumb feet.

Tom put the heater a too-generous distance from the chair. "You need to check your sugar and write it down once more before bedtime, and again in the morning. Just write the number in on this line," he said, highlighting the place with a pencil. "We need to keep close track of this." He placed her glucose monitor and the lancets on a tray table next to her chair. "If this don't work, you can't stay by yourself."

Lacy fixed crackers with peanut butter, and orange slices, wrapped them in baggies, placed a couple within easy reach and left the others in the refrigerator. She reminded Imogene about the frozen dinners in the freezer, showed her how to put them in the microwave and which button to push to have an instant, nutritious, warm and sensible meal.

Would it be any worse at Shannondale?

"We're gonna head home," Tom said. He looked uneasy. "Anything else you can think of we need to do?" He checked the equipment on her tray, moved the remote to the TV within easy reach, as if he was stalling.

"I reckon not," Imogene said.

"And you know how to reach us," Tom said.

"I have both of your work numbers wrote down by the phone in case I need something," Imogene said.

Their boots scraped on the back steps. She listened to Lacy chatter until her voice cut off abruptly when the truck door slammed shut. Imogene watched out the window as Tom backed down the drive. The top of her dining room table glowed under the streetlamp when they drove under it.

"I'll just sit here and check my blood sugar and look out the window and eat out of these little plastic baggies," she said as the red taillights disappeared around the corner at the end of the street.

*　　*　　*

Imogene clicked the remote control to the only station her television could reach. "Low tonight in the teens without the wind chill, and there's a slight chance of snow in the higher elevations," droned the weatherman from somewhere in Knoxville. The television screen distorted his body like those carnival mirrors that make even handsome people look grotesque. She switched off the TV and listened to the night sounds. The wind moaned softly outside. A tree limb scratched at the house where it hung low over the roof.

She unplugged the electric space heater, then sat on the edge of her new bed to catch her breath. She was weaker than she thought. The dining room disappeared as the heater's glow faded. She fluffed her pillow, snuggled under the covers. She missed her bed, hers and Carl's. She struggled onto her left side, touched the top handrail. The bars were cool. Moonlight trickled through the kitchen window, illuminating the door to the garage. Carl was waiting for her, if she could only get there. She tried to pull herself up, shaking the rails, hard. The rattling bed mocked her.

REFLECTIONS

She often walked about her house naked, moving from room to room, admiring herself in her mirrors, stiffening her spine, and studying the firm contour of her belly still flat at the age of forty-five. She wore her black hair coiled in a French twist, low on the back of her neck. Long necklaces looped around her throat and fell out of sight between breasts hidden but not concealed by exotic, loose fitting robes. She bathed twice daily. She smelled perpetually of soap, shampoo and perfume. She exercised sparingly and meditated every morning and night. She painted in oils, read poetry, played the piano. This was Ada before she found the lump.

She discovered it by accident, appearing while she was admiring the image of her body and the foliage of an oak tree in her yard, both reflected in one of her living room mirrors. Posing, partly for herself and partly for the boys she knew played in that tree, she had reached upward to remove a silver comb from her hair and twisted to watch it cascade down across her shoulders toward a rose tattooed in the small of her back.

It mocked her from the mirror, first catching only the corner of her eye. She pirouetted back to face it, arms still raised, hands still playing in her hair. It bulged again, painlessly from the upper part of her right breast, puckering the skin and pulling her nipple up in an ugly angle. She dropped her arms. The breast regained its smooth, seductive, symmetric contour, a mirror image of its healthy mate. She kneaded the area frantically, confirming the foreign hardness there. She marked its edges, mentally comparing its size to that of a marble.

She was suddenly ashamed of her nakedness. She turned toward the window, hoping no witnesses lurked in the tree. She scooped a silk robe from the floor, clutched it to her chest and cowered down the hallway to her bedroom. Curtains drawn, lights dimmed, she tried to meditate, tried to force her mind to think pure thoughts. Instead, eyes closed, she visualized the lump removed from her body, laying on a rock in the back yard, covered with red ants, each taking a bite, carrying it off piece by piece until it was gone.

She reached for her telephone, thought better of it and resolved to try to meditate again. Her mind raced faster, from one thought to another, one time to another, one place to another. She reached for the phone again, this time punching the numbers. She sighed when she heard it ring. She slammed the phone down when a female voice answered. She clutched her throat, breathing heavily, a chilly sweat oozing from her pores. She'd have to call in the morning, have to ask Melissa to make her a work-in appointment to see him like she was just another patient. She blushed at the thought.

Dr. Corless had been her mother's doctor while she died. He had just moved to town after his own father passed away. Ada was attracted to him by the way he talked to her, the way he explained things, the way he prepared her for what would happen next in her mother's journey through the end of life.

She felt like she had known him all her life. They both had grown up in Oak Grove, both moved away, both returned very different people. While Ada was five years older, she claimed to remember him when they were in school. She assured her mother that they had nurtured a friendship that was special, and that fate had chosen him for her doctor. She told her mother that they kept in touch while she was in college and after, when she was traveling around the country with strangers in a multi-colored Volkswagen van. She was almost certain she remembered conversations with him though details eluded her.

She had sensed something spiritual between herself and Dr. Corless. The feeling was so strong that she had dispensed with formality within minutes of their first meeting about her mother. She had called him by his nick name, Ike, short for Isaac, a presumptuous move in a town where, as the only doctor, he was a near deity. She had convinced herself that he could not extend such kindness, such extraordinary compassion to someone for whom he did not have a deep and abiding emotional appeal.

She positioned herself close to him when he examined her mother in the office or when he visited her at home. She would lean on his arm when he tried to leave, beg his forgiveness for being so weak, and imagine the fire that raged in him for her.

Ada knew how it felt to be wanted. When she walked down Main Street admiring her image in the store windows, she could see the reflection of rheumy eyed, whittling men studying her figure as she passed them in a flimsy sun dress. She assumed Ike was just as enchanted.

She was hurt when Ike didn't come to her mother's funeral. She was relieved, even forgave him, when she read his return address on the envelope of a sympathy card, but disappointed again to find that it only had his signature. She had hoped for a few lines personalizing their status as comrades-at-arms in the care of her mother or something to acknowledge their status as fellow sufferers since they had each lost a parent. But after introspection, she realized that it would be unseemly for him to expose such a relationship so soon after being involved in the care of a patient's family member. Why else would he avoid her?

She had waited. After plenty of time for small minded, small-town people to accept the idea that Ike was in love with the beautiful daughter of a patient, he had still not called. Three months after her mother died, Ada called his office leaving a message that she had a question about her mother's death certificate. She had been so confident of their need to communicate, his willingness to talk if given the opportunity, that she had not even formulated a real question.

He had returned her call in the middle of the afternoon. The annoyance that simmered in Ike's voice when he found there was no reason for the call surprised Ada.

"I'm really busy," he said. "I have a waiting room full of people to see." She had chided him about being a workaholic hoping to hear him chuckle and carry on with his end of the conversation. Instead, he had hung up without answering her.

"Well, you should have known better than to call during office hours," she said as she replaced the phone in its cradle. He didn't answer any of the many messages she left for him after that, despite her accusations to the receptionist that she was not passing them along to him.

A few evenings later, she called him at home, wine glass in her hand, legs curled under her, lights turned low, wearing nothing but a gold ankle chain and candlelight.

"Hello," she said when he picked up the telephone. She let the tip of her tongue caress the rim of her wineglass, as if he could see her, as if they were sitting head-to-head across a table in a crowded restaurant, alone in the masses, whispering secrets. He hadn't answered, had placed the receiver back into the cradle so firmly that she thought he must have been called away to an emergency. But when she called again after an hour, his machine answered for him. Over several days, she left him messages, at first seductive, then furious, then pleading. Then she mailed long letters. Even the first one returned, unopened.

Desperate, she had scheduled an appointment, had told the receptionist that she needed to see Dr. Corless about a persistent headache. When Ike came into the exam room that day, he had barely acknowledged her, had not even mentioned her mother's death. She could detect no compassion, no sympathy in his bearing. He just sat on his stainless-steel stool, all the way across the room, back full against the wall, reading the new patient questionnaire. She realized now that she had not completed it as honestly as she should have. In her past medical history, she had listed several childhood illnesses but omitted two prolonged admissions to a psychiatric hospital that had occurred during a very exhausting period in her life. She had hoped he would consider it humorous where she had described in her social history a fictional fascination with snakes. She should have limited her completion of the family history section to the genealogy of heart disease and cancer that was her legacy. Instead, after she had listed no siblings and no children of her own, she expounded on her conscious choice to forego childbearing because of global, social and economic concerns for future generations. Dr. Corless had studied the form, then looked at her over the rim of his glasses. She could feel his skepticism vibrate across the room.

She had hoped for that visit, the headache visit, to be a revelation to Ike, an opportunity for him to confront his feelings for her. She wanted him to understand what she had realized during her mother's dying, that in her loss they had ministered to each other, that they were two parts of a whole, two halves of the same story. She had rehearsed the way to say these things in front of her mirrors, had practiced quivering her chin, pictured herself collapsing into his arms at the point where he apologized for the unanswered phone calls, the unopened letters. But his detached, professional manner had confused her. She had faltered, then panicked, then abandoned her plan. She had tried to talk to Dr. Corless about her headaches as if they were real, the way she imagined a headache would feel.

"I have headaches, daily, but I feel no pain from them," she said. "I acknowledge their presence but without experiencing discomfort. I think it is similar to looking out the window and seeing it rain. I see the rain and experience its presence, but I don't get wet. Most of the time my headaches don't hurt, but sometimes they do." She winced inwardly as she heard herself conclude. "They are not like the headaches normal people have."

Her mind had raced. She had watched him, worried that he might now be attracted to her because of the vulnerability her headaches granted her, then she feared a relationship based on disease would not be healthy or lasting. She blushed again as she remembered her words, "They are not like the headaches normal people have."

Melissa, Ike's clinic nurse, had mercifully knocked on the exam room door, had told Ike that he had a phone call from another doctor. After he excused himself, Ada had gathered her things, tiptoed down the empty hallway and exited through a side door. It was a relief, for a few days, when he didn't call to ask her why she had left so quickly. But after a week, when he still hadn't called, his transparent lack of concern caused her to paint a likeness of the oak tree as reflected in her mirror, entirely in shades of gray and black.

She settled back on her pillows again. These things happened a year ago. Maybe he won't remember. Besides, this lump is not imaginary like the headaches. And she needed a doctor and he was the only one in town. Reassured that she had no reason to be embarrassed, she resumed her efforts to meditate. She finally gave up and slept poorly the rest of the night.

Melissa almost did not let her make the appointment. "Dr. Corless has no openings for a new patient today," she said.

Ada reminded her that she was not a new patient.

"Is it an emergency?"

"I found a lump in my breast," she said, and surprised herself by adding, "My mother died of breast cancer, and I am terrified." She shuddered. The words were even more frightening when spoken.

She waited for several minutes while the telephone played country music from the only radio station in Oak Grove. Melissa came back on the line. "Come in at noon. He'll see you during the lunch break."

"Thank you, Melissa," she said and hung up the phone. She wondered if this was a concession, a message, a sign that he did care. Her spirits buoyed until her fingers stole under her gown and palpated the lump.

She arrived at the clinic early, sat in the waiting room crossing and uncrossing her legs, picking at her fingernails, taking inventory of her purse. She flipped through the stack of magazines, settling on one that contained an article documenting that all diseases result from a build-up of noxious poisons created as waste from normal tissues. Before she could read it, Melissa called from the entrance to the clinical area.

"Ada. You can come on back now." Ada tilted her head down, avoiding Melissa's gaze when she rose to follow her to the exam room. The place was cool, white, and somber, the way she imagined the inside of a mausoleum. It smelled of menthol, just the way it did on visits when she had accompanied her mother. She couldn't associate a smell with the headache appointment. Ada wondered what Ike had written in her record about that visit.

He entered the room, assumed his position on the stool, backing it up close to the wall where he could support his back.

"This is not about headaches," she said.

He sat, his face expressionless.

"I found a lump in my breast, Dr. Corless. I didn't know who to call. You're the only doctor here in Oak Grove and even if you weren't, I have so much respect for how you treated my mother...I know this is awkward for you, but it is for me too, and I want you to examine me and tell me what I need to do. Even if it's to go to someone else, tell me what to do."

He stood up, hesitated for a minute, then folded her chart and left it on the stool. He handed her a gown.

"Put this on," he said. "Just undress from the waist up." He stepped outside the exam room and stood by the door while she changed. When Ike returned, Ada was surprised to see that Melissa accompanied him.

Ike examined Ada without speaking. She watched his brow furrow when she lifted her arm to demonstrate the puckering of her nipple, noted his frown when she directed his attention to the dimpled skin near her armpit. His hand felt warm on her breast as he found and rolled the mass under his fingers. She felt a pinch when his wedding band caught her skin. She was instantly saddened by this reminder, wondered if they might have established a more meaningful relationship had this third party not hindered them.

He seemed to soften. He smiled his reassuring smile, the one she recognized from her mother's illness. She felt emboldened and tried to engage him in a dialogue about the cause of the nodule and her proposed solution to it. She watched his smile disappear.

"I think this is a cancer, not just a nodule," he said. "And I know it is not a vitamin deficiency or a dietary problem." The word cancer, even more alarming when he said it, had a lot more negative connotations than she was prepared to deal with at a time when she felt so vulnerable. She didn't push the issue.

Ike left the room to allow her to dress. When he returned, he had written instructions regarding an appointment he had made for her with a surgeon in Knoxville. He had impatiently stuffed the card in her purse when she declined to accept it directly from his hand to hers. She tried to explain to him that her acceptance of the card, rather than just discovering it in her purse, implied her acceptance of this lump as a malignancy. It was important, even if it proved to be so, that she not accept it so readily. He sighed and started to write in her chart.

"I'm sorry I bothered you." She gathered her things and stood to leave. "Thank you for your time." She did not wait to see if he answered. On her way out, she snatched the magazine with the article about noxious waste from the hands of an old man who was reading it. She stuffed it into her purse with the appointment card.

"He is just as closed-minded as any minion of the medical industry," she announced to the people in the waiting room before she slammed the clinic door behind her. "He is certainly not the same compassionate man who cared for my mother," she continued as she marched down the sidewalk toward home.

But later, after she had time to reflect, she realized that he could not deal with his feelings for her and this lump simultaneously. Because of the threat to their relationship, she reasoned, he must have viewed it as malignant whether or not it was actually a cancer. "That explains a lot," she said.

She read the magazine article, making notes in the margins regarding ways to incorporate the program of coffee enemas, purifying fruits and positive thinking into her treatment plan. She used the appointment card to mark the start of another article advising that she drink green tea three times daily. She consumed glass after glass of water with a lemon rind in each to titrate the acid level in her blood and let her body's poisons filter out through her kidneys. She resolved to look up the word titrate when she happened to be near a dictionary, but as promised, thought she already felt a little less alkaline, a little healthier after only one day on her program.

After several months, she stood in front of her mirror to judge her progress, her clothes draped to reveal only her right chest and shoulder. She was disappointed to find the reflection of a sad face and an asymmetric, swollen breast that had developed the appearance of an orange peel.

Ada then persuaded herself that her theory was the opposite of the truth, a mirror image of reality. This unwanted part of her, this proliferating clump of cells was not the result of a buildup of noxious cellular waste products after all. It was, rather, a group of cells that lacked something. In effect, she argued, the rest of her had deprived this nodule. The original cell that went bad had been the runt of the litter, had grown to compensate, had become inappropriately strong because of the bullying by the healthy parts of her. That is why it had thrived on her program of cleansing and purging. Only this theory explained how a part of her could rebel against the whole.

She swallowed vitamin C tablets until diarrhea forced her to stop. Vitamin E capsules left her mouth feeling greasy and her stomach nauseous. She took Vitamin A pills until her vision started to blur. She pulverized fruits and vegetables and drank a glass full every other waking hour. She added dairy products to a diet previously vegan, then removed them again.

After a few more months, she had to fashion a crude sling to support the weight of her right arm, now swollen to twice its normal size. She padded her armpit with a throw pillow to absorb the pain that stabbed her shoulder with every step. She slept with her arm propped on cushions, her wrist on her forehead, an unconscious signal of hopelessness and despair. She wondered, sometimes, if her own vicious thoughts had complicated her recovery.

She stormed Ike's clinic the last time she saw him. She walked into the sitting area full of worried people, signed her name left-handed to the long list of waiting patients and sat down. The receptionist had looked at her, pulled her chart and put it at the front of the stack without saying a word. Melissa escorted her back to an exam room, her nostrils flaring a little with what Ada knew was the musty odor of cancer that followed her like a cloud.

She watched Ike study her swollen hand while she talked, felt his gaze on her for the first time since her mother's death. She saw him wince when she unwrapped her arm and uncovered her breast. She detected panic in her face reflected in the luminous blue of his eyes.

"You didn't see the surgeon?" He flipped back through her chart. "That was a year ago." He looked up at her again, disbelieving. "Why did you ignore this?"

Ada replied that she had not ignored it, in fact, had thought of little else for the past twelve months.

She watched him squirm on his stool, listened to him telling her in stuttering, short sentences that she had missed a "window of opportunity," that now her condition was incurable and the only thing medicine could offer her was comfort. Melissa stood through the harangue like a doe-eyed witness at a murder trial.

Ike made her another appointment, this time with a radiation therapist. He wrote her a prescription for oxycodone, assuming that if she was not hurting bad enough to need it, she would be soon. She accepted this prescription from him directly, as a tangible expression of his compassion and concern for her, noting that a pale band of skin marked the place where his wedding ring used to be.

"I'm sorry," she said.

She thought Ike started to reach for her, to put his hand around her shoulder to commiserate with her. She understood when he didn't.

She used this appointment card to mark the book of Job in the Bible she had resolved to read. She renewed her efforts, incorporating nostrums that she ordered from advertisements in magazines, catalogs and on television. At first, she convinced herself that the mass got smaller, that the swelling in her arm was receding. Then, in a flash of intellectual honesty, she took solace that it had not grown. When it broke through the skin, pouring its putrid contents down her side, she rationalized the smelly drainage as an expulsion of poisons occurring as the result of her cleansing program. When the stench of the ulcer overwhelmed her perfume, she mixed healing vegetable pastes and smeared them onto the yawning wound several times daily.

Ada shuffled painfully through her house, a pink terry cloth bathrobe hanging loose from her shoulder, the front moist with a mixture of pus and poultice. Stacks of old magazines and newspapers covered the floor, the chairs, and the tables. A dank, mildewed smell permeated every room. Her mirrors stood shrouded in bed sheets and quilts to hide her reflection.

A circulating fan, straining to move the stagnant air, fanned the sheet away from the living room mirror as she hobbled by it. The image of the oak tree appeared, its naked gnarled trunk stripped of its summer foliage, skinny limbs reaching upward, a caricature of the hideous and the lonely. Ada traced the reflected image of the tree with the fingers of her good hand, first the limbs, then downward along the trunk. She knelt by the mirror, watched as her image settled slowly to the floor and landed softly. She turned her eyes away from the mirror and looked out the window toward the dying tree. She cried and cried.

AVY'S PLACE

Darryl let the truck engine idle while the radio played sad country songs, and the heater worked just hard enough to keep off the chill. The night was so clear that he could hear the whine of tractor-trailer tires on the highway miles away. He leaned backward savoring the warmth the leather upholstery had absorbed from the heat of a September sun. He rubbed his chest with his fingertips.

This was his retreat. He felt out of place in the hospital. The young nurses made him feel self-conscious. The old ones made him feel inadequate. The doctor, a high school classmate named Ike Corless, reminded him of paths others took to other places, forced him to review the path he had taken here. His boots, his jeans, the pack of Marlboros peeking from the pocket of his flannel shirt did not belong in those sterile surroundings. He needed the outdoors, the sun above him, a breeze blowing around him, a trowel in one hand and a brick in the other.

He needed to talk to Ike again to reassure himself that Avy was doing as expected, that she was dying comfortably. Darryl was always misreading the signs. When he thought Avy was sleeping a lot, Ike said she might be entering a "light coma." Darryl thought her furrowed brow meant she was trying to talk to him. He had hovered with his ear over her lips for almost an hour until a nurse gave Avy an injection of something for pain that made her forehead smooth again.

The chaplain had tried to help him understand. He explained that the doctors and nurses were now just treating the essence of Avy, keeping her body subdued while her soul wrestled free.

What the hell does that mean, Darryl wondered while he shook hands and thanked the man.

He had waited as long as he could, waited so long he felt like he was going to explode. Like a diver, he needed to resurface occasionally, had to sit in his diving bell in the hospital parking lot to avoid suffocating. The nurse promised she would find him if the doctor appeared while he was outside.

Darryl inhaled and exhaled several times, fighting the smothering sensation of panic sweeping over him. He looked up at the sky, so clear that it made the world look colder. He listened as the wind rustled through the leaves in a park across the street. He had noticed earlier that they were changing colors. When she was healthy, Avy raked the leaves in their yard as fast as they fell.

He gathered himself to go back inside, breathed in deep a few more times, each inhalation longer and deeper than before. He stepped down from the cab, locked the door and walked across the parking lot to the hospital entrance. He turned toward the glass sliding doors, slipped through the suffocating medicinal smell of the lobby, then rode the chrome elevator until it crested on the second floor, all in one breath.

His work boots scuffed at the shiny tile surface of the corridor. He walked past the nursing station and nodded to the ward clerk who looked up briefly and smiled. He hesitated, then opened the door to the room where Avy rested. Moonlight filtered through the window across her bed. Her hands were folded on her stomach, fingers intertwined, as white and detailed as the cheap figurine of praying hands she kept on the mantle in their living room.

She had told him she wanted to die at home. She felt more comfortable there, she said, surrounded by her things. No matter how hard he tried, he could not humiliate her with the things he had to do to keep her there. Once, while trying to force hands that were better suited to handling cement and cinderblocks to change her wet diaper, out of the corner of his eye he saw that tears had pooled in hers. He could not force himself to place a suppository in her rectum, no matter how hard she wretched. He coaxed her to swallow pills long after she was too weak to do it safely, long after he knew he would find them later, half-dissolved under her tongue, or on her pillow. The time that prompted his moving her to the hospice, she had choked on water he had her try to sip from a spoon. She coughed and gasped the hour it took the home nurse to reach them from where she lived on the other side of the ridge.

"Avy needs more care than you can give her by yourself, Darryl," the nurse said. "I think we should move her to where she can have skilled care."

He struggled with the decision, worried that Avy would become bitter toward him. He surrendered after he realized she didn't know where she was anyway.

Darryl pulled a rocking chair into the moonlight between the window and Avy's bed. He remembered an autumn night when they sat together on Marion Ridge looking down on Oak Grove. He remembered how she had rested her head on his chest while they looked at the flickering lights scattered randomly in the valley.

"I want to stay in this place," she whispered.

"I'll come back," he said.

"No," she said. "Not here in Oak Grove. I want to be here, where I can hear your heart beat, hear you whisper, feel your breath when it blows over my face. This place."

"I'll come back," he said again.

Later, when he sat in the dark and listened to raindrops slapping on jungle leaves, he would tilt his head down and imagine he could smell her hair. When he saw the flash of rifle fire in the distance, he would remember the lights in the valley. When his rifle squad walked into an ambush, when time spasmed and the blue sky was still hidden by a pink mist that settled gently on the jungle foliage, when the odor of burning flesh overwhelmed his memory of Avy's perfume, when Darryl woke in a ditch with a fellow marine's head resting on his chest, he thought of Avy and how her head had rested exactly where this soldier died.

While Darryl was recovering at the naval hospital in Bethesda, he would lie for hours, eyes closed, feeling the stare of strangers wearing white uniforms, hearing them whisper clinical secrets about him. Long after his visible wounds had disappeared, he would rub absently at his chest, look into distance, like he was studying something far away.

Things were not the same when he got home. Avy had bargained with God for his safe return, joined a little Pentecostal church that met in a renovated house hidden in the byways near Oak Grove. She read her Bible daily, prayed without ceasing, lived a year of quiet reflection with the assurance that if she did these things, God would spare his life. Darryl had watched young men die because of old men's decisions and grew to doubt His existence. At night when the pressure of darkness compressed the volatile mix of memories and emotions that he still carried, she held his head to her chest so he could listen for her heartbeat, be soothed by her voice, and feel her warm breath blowing over him.

Her inability to speak now made him regret the many times they could have talked and didn't. She hadn't told him about the mass in her breast. He had noticed she couldn't walk from the house to the mailbox without resting, noticed the outline of her face, gaunt and pale, and how her clothes hung loose on her, like draperies. When he took her to the clinic, the cancer had already invaded half way through her chest toward her heart, filling one lung with a viscous, malignant fluid.

It had been four months since their first visit with Dr. Corless. He had examined Avy, then looked at Darryl with his own thousand-mile stare, as if he was wondering how two people could have shared a bed without acknowledging this concretion in her breast.

She hadn't spoken to anyone for two days. Ike had told him that Avy had definitely entered a coma from which it was not likely she would return. He encouraged Darryl to talk as if he expected her to answer.

"You never know what they are hearing," he said. "Sometimes people wake up, and it's surprising what they remember."

Darryl had talked to her, seizing on the glimmer of hope the doctor had accidentally kindled in him. She smiled once. He was almost sure of that. She had gripped his hand when he touched hers, searched his calluses, caressed the stump of his missing index finger. The nurses smiled when he told them. The doctor nodded wisely, put his hand on Darryl's shoulder and said, "I'm sorry you're having such a hard time." Darryl decided not to mention it to the chaplain.

He leaned over, touched her chest, felt her heartbeat once, and then again, knowing that the ripple of this pulse, which had started in some ancestor an eternity ago, would end with Avy. They had no children. He took her hand again, to see if she squeezed back.

"Avy, I'm gonna go back to the house tonight." He paused and watched the lacy network of blood vessels visible in the thin skin of her eyelids. There was no panic, no searching gaze, no flutter of recognition. "I need to clean up a little, shave, maybe pay some bills. I bet the yard's a mess, too." He paused for a second, smiling a tepid smile. "You've fell down on your duties as the yard boy." He watched her face looking for a sign that she appreciated his humor. "I'll be back." He rubbed his chin with its three-day growth of facial hair, as if to show her that he wasn't making up an excuse to go home.

He waited a moment longer, stroking Avy's hair, still dark, luxuriant, and so heavy it seemed to anchor her head to the pillow. She had not cut it since she joined the Pentecostals. She told Darryl that the Bible said a woman's hair was her glory. He never argued, never challenged the verses she quoted him. He wondered if she had declined chemotherapy for fear of losing both. Outside, the moon went behind a cloud, darkening the room for a few seconds. As it emerged on the other side, the light filtered back across her face.

Darryl picked up a jar of homemade jelly that he had brought her. He felt silly about it now. She hadn't eaten in days, and a jar of jelly wasn't likely to change that. He had needed an offering. It embarrassed him to realize that the only thing he could bring her was something she had made for him. He shut the door quietly behind him and stopped at the nursing station.

"I'm goin' back to our place for tonight."

"Thanks, Mr. Delaney. We'll take good care of her."

"Do you think she'll be OK? It'll take me a half hour to get back to Oak Grove from here. I don't want her to be by herself, if she..., when she..."

He felt his throat tighten. As much as he hated all the substitute words and phrases he had learned this month, he couldn't make himself say the word "dies." He once overheard a nurse calling someone on the phone, saying that a woman had "expired," like she was a magazine whose subscription had run out. He cringed when they used the word "terminal." Every time he heard it, he thought of lonely places, like a bus station with two people saying goodbye in the rain.

"Her blood pressure and pulse have been stable for the past 24 hours. I think you're safe. Go home. Get some rest."

"If she changes..."

"I have your phone number. Try not to worry."

He stood awkwardly, at once feeling guilty and relieved that this stranger had given her blessing to his going home. "Here." He handed the jar of strawberry preserves to the nurse. "You take these. She ain't goin' to eat, an' I don't want to carry 'em back home."

The nurse took the jar and smiled at him. "Go home, Mr. Delaney. I'll take good care of her. I promise."

The hospital smell, much stronger in the hallway than in Avy's room, caused the smothering sensation to settle over him in earnest. He rode the elevator down, walked quickly across the lobby, knowing that if he could hold his breath another thirty feet, he would breathe the pure night air of an East Tennessee autumn.

Darryl steered his Dodge pickup slowly along the valley road. He put the truck in low gear before making the turn to climb the long hill that led to their driveway. He stopped and removed a three-day accumulation of letters and parcels from a brick mailbox so ponderous it could have marked the entry to the courthouse. The crunching sound the balloon tires made on the gravel reassured him.

He stood in the dark, studying the house. The moon highlighted some of Darryl's best masonry work. Brick bolstered the ancient frame structure he and Avy had shared for the past three decades. He'd built brick sidewalks, brick fences, a brick patio. The workshop and garage had brickwork in a pattern to match the house.

He walked into the kitchen, remembered the times he had listened as she stood washing dishes, singing, "Amazing Grace." He moved to the living room and saw the outline of her body in the chair where she sat to read her Bible. Avy's glasses rested on the table next to it, like she had just removed them and stood up to stroll toward the hereafter.

He came to their bedroom and sat on her side of the bed. His jeans scuffed the spread. He folded it back and rubbed his gnarled hands on the sheet. His calluses caught on the clean linens. He remembered the nights when he had slept with his back to her, waking to the weight of her gaze on his neck, knowing that she worried about his soul.

He moved to the screen-enclosed porch outside their bedroom. Darkness always magnified his fears, amplified his senses. He could hear things in the woods not audible during the day, frogs croaking, crickets chirping. He saw the silhouette of a deer he knew would have been invisible in daylight.

He sat in his chair all night, rocking silently, thinking his own dark thoughts, wondering about his purpose, his place in a world without Avy.

"The dying process is the hardest part," the chaplain said, "because you and Avy have to share it."

Darryl didn't answer.

"There is a whole set of other feelings one has when the dying stops and the death occurs," he said. "You will grieve for a time, then things will normalize. You should prepare to move on with your life. Let Avy's death mark a time of new beginnings."

Darryl remembered the war, remembered his buddy's dying process compressed into a span of less than a minute. That had never normalized. Death lasts forever in the minds of those left behind.

He felt better when the first drops of burnt orange filtered through the veil of morning fog. He listened for other signs that day was near. As if in preparation for their morning devotions, the wildlife stopped moving, chirping and singing, leaving the world still and quiet for a few minutes. Through some acoustic miracle, he could hear irreverent fishermen talking and laughing on the river, a half-mile away, their words muffled beyond recognition by the fog and foliage. He strained to hear the first faint rumbling of the 5:05 a.m. Southern Pacific freight train before it exploded through the valley, clacking and clattering on its way from Knoxville to Chattanooga. That noisy climax always reassured him. It meant that he and Avy had survived another night.

The phone rang. Darryl jerked to his feet, leaving the empty chair rocking behind him.

"You need to come back," the nurse said. "But don't rush. There's no need to rush." Darryl held the phone at his side and tried to breathe normally. His mind swirled. He walked back to the porch and listened to the noise of the locomotive fade into the distance.

CHARLIE BENSON SEES THE OCEAN

Charlie Benson was way past knee walking drunk when he fell and banged his head on the corner of his bed. That afternoon, his foreman had laid him off from the best job he ever had, making union money at the TVA as a carpenter's assistant. He'd cashed his check at the Blockhouse on the way home and bought as much Thunderbird wine as he could carry, then drank himself to sleep in the bedroom in the back of his trailer. When the urge to pee woke him, he stumbled to the tiny bathroom adjacent to his bed. The last thing he remembered was the view of Roan Mountain through his bedroom window as he fell on the way back.

He woke with a headache like he'd never had before and pain that seared through his feet into his ankles. He smelled the odor of something burning and assumed the worst. "I ain't dead yet," he yelled. "You can't take me there till I'm dead." He pulled his knees up to his chest.

He felt a cool damp washcloth on his feet. *This can't be hell*, he thought. *There's no water down there.*

"Who are you," he asked. "I ain't dead yet…" His voice trailed off. He struggled again, pulled his feet up higher, away from the pain, away from the flames.

"Amy," the owner of the hands said. He couldn't make out her face.

"You're a devil girl," he screamed. "I know what you're doing. I ain't dead yet." The yelling made his head hurt worse. He lost consciousness for a minute.

When he revived a little, he heard a male voice say, "He's probably in DTs. Run out of money to buy liquor."

Charlie craned his neck back and looked up. He could see the vague outline of a round, red face floating well above a huge belly. It kept changing shapes, like those mirrors at the Marion County fair that make your head look too big, or too small, or you don't have arms, or something.

He could make out the girl's shape now, too. She wore ragged jeans and a sweatshirt. Her arms hugged her chest like she was cold. Her tongue loved her lips. It kept sneaking out there to touch them. For a moment, Charlie wanted to lick them, too, but he remembered who she was and where she was trying to lure him. He wondered if the flickering tongue was forked like a snake's.

"My name's Slim," the man said. Amy said something back that Charlie couldn't understand. Slim continued, "…part-time paramedic and a part-time deputy sheriff for Oak Grove."

Charlie thought Slim was talking to him.

"I know who you are," he said. "You're so fat everybody calls you Slim." He looked at the end of the bed.

"He ain't changed since high school," Slim said.

Amy and Slim leaned over Charlie. They looked like one body with two heads. Slim talked non-stop while Amy's tongue flicked in and out like it was sensing the air, preparing to strike. Every pounding heartbeat felt like someone was swirling an ice pick in his brain. Slim covered him with a blanket that had a Marion County EMS logo on it. Charlie vomited over the side of the bed as the world faded away to silence.

Charlie woke on clean sheets, propped up on pillows. A skinny girl stood next to his bed eating cafeteria food off the tray on his over-the-bed table. There was something vaguely familiar about her.

"Who the hell are you?"

"Look at you," she said. "One week in a coma and you wake up cussin'."

Charlie didn't speak.

She moved a little, to let him focus on her.

"You ain't a nurse," he said. "Not in them jeans."

"At least you ain't brain damaged." She dropped the peas back on the plate. "I'm Amy. I saved your life, so you better be nice to me."

"I don't remember that," he said.

She waited for several seconds, as if debating whether or not to share.

"It's a long story," she said.

"I got time."

She paused again, as if organizing her thoughts. "I was hitchhiking," she said. "I got a ride with a man who told me he was going to Knoxville."

She hesitated again and swirled her spoon in the mash potatoes. "Turns out he's your neighbor...lives in that shack down the road from you."

"Scraggle Mahoney?"

"Scraggle fits. He needed a haircut and a good bath."

"He's a pervert."

She put a bit of the mashed potatoes on the spoon, then dumped them and loaded the peas again.

"I figured out he wasn't going to Knoxville. I told him I wanted out. He kept saying he wanted to show me something."

"He's a pervert," Charlie said again. He looked at the spoon, now loaded and aimed at his face. The melody to "That's How I got to Memphis" ran through his mind. He loved to strum his guitar along with that song. "How'd you get away?"

"When he parked, I just got out and started walking."

Charlie studied Amy. Scraggle spent most of his time chain smoking cigarettes and watching porn on his VCR. He couldn't walk ten feet without getting short of breath. He couldn't have chased her if he tried.

"I looked back once. He looked like I'd hurt his feelings."

"Perverts don't have feelings. What was you thinking?"

"I wanted to get to Myrtle Beach," she answered. "My mom's new boyfriend was getting too friendly and I was getting in her way." Her voice dropped almost to a whisper. "I was goin' to look for one of them summertime jobs waitin' tables." She studied the napkin on Charlie's tray. "People say I look like a college girl when I dress up a little."

"You don't sound like no college girl," Charlie said.

"It just took a ninth grade education to save your pitiful life," she said. She resumed torturing the peas and potatoes.

"Plus, it's September."

"Be nice."

Charlie relaxed a little and leaned his head back on his pillow. He'd heard enough, but Amy continued. "It was real dark. I wouldn't of noticed your trailer except when I walked by, I saw flames shoot up in one of the windows. It was so sudden, I wasn't sure it was real. I ran over and looked in your window and saw your heater had just set fire to your bed spread." She put the spoon on the plate and wiped her hands on Charlie's sheet. "So I just let myself in and saved your life."

Charlie tried to shrug his right shoulder, then tried to flex the fingers. "My arm's gone to sleep," he said.

"It ain't asleep," she said. "You had blood clog on your brain from where you hit your head. Doc Corless says you same as had a stroke."

Charlie wiggled his feet. The right one was a little sluggish, but he could manage. He tried his hand again, barely got the fingers to grip.

"Where am I," he asked.

"The hospital."

"Any particular one?"

"University."

"Did they fly me over here?" Charlie had never flown anywhere, so if he had, he would have been disappointed to not have known it.

"Naw, you didn't rate the helicopter. They sent you in an ambulance." She stuck the peas in her mouth and chewed slowly, as if considering how best to continue the story. "The emergency doctor thought you was just drunk. He tried to make Slim take you to jail." She loaded the spoon again. "Slim told him you'd had a seizure on the way in, so it was against regulations."

Charlie was pretty sure he'd had a seizure in the drunk tank before. No one had paid much attention to it.

"The emergency doctor called Doc Corless to admit you to the hospital. Doc saw right off there was something more than just being drunk goin' on. He yelled something about a 'blown pupil.' Next thing I knew he'd shaved the side of your head, drilled a hole in your skull and drained a blood clog."

Charlie rubbed the side of his head. There was a bald patch, and a sore spot that felt like it had staples in it.

"And you was standing right there," Charlie said. "Bullshit." He closed his eyes and imagined someone with a power drill to his skull. He'd had a few headaches that felt like that.

"The neurosurgeon said Doc had prob'ly done a million of those when he was in Vietnam. He was real nice. He thinks I'm your fiancée, by the way, in case anybody asks."

156

Charlie looked around him. "How long have I been here?" he asked.

"Long enough that they're talking about sending you to the old folks home." Amy had another spoon full of peas aimed at his mouth. "You ain't talked in days. They think you've got permanent brain damage."

Charlie felt nauseous again. "I ain't ready for that," he said.

"The home?"

"The peas," he said. "You finish 'em. Looks like you're 'bout to anyway."

"Thanks," she said. "I am kinda hungry."

Amy ate like a machine. She finished the peas before moving to the potatoes, and finished the potatoes before she sliced the meatloaf. "They send you a tray three times a day. It seems like a sin to waste it," she said.

How can she be this skinny when she eats like that, Charlie wondered.

"Kind of puts me in a bind," she continued. "As long as you're out of your head, I get to eat pretty high on the hog. You get better, and I got nothing again. Funny ain't it? The way things even out."

"So are they gonna put me in the home, or not?"

She dabbed at her mouth with a paper napkin before she cut a sliver of cherry pie. "This'd probably be too rich for you," she said. She loaded it on her fork and hesitated. "You want to try a bite?" she asked as she put it in her mouth.

"Are they sending me to Shannondale?" Charlie asked again.

"Nope," she said. "I threw a fit. I told them I'm taking you home with me."

"Where's that?"

"Your trailer," she said. "I don't have any place, so it kinda balances out."

*   *   *

Everything Charlie liked about Amy was right there leaning against the doorframe; long legs, cutoff jeans, worn out flip flops, the way she would tie a shoelace around her ankle and wear it like a bracelet. What he didn't like was what she had just told him.

"*We* ain't havin' no baby," Charlie said. He stubbed his cigarette out on the side of his coffee cup, hitched his chair around as best he could with his partially paralyzed right arm and his guitar on his lap. He liked to hold it, even though he couldn't strum any more.

Amy's blonde hair dangled over her left eye. It made her squint like Charlie was a reflection too painful to face. "Well, I am, and you're the only one I've been with." She brushed the lock of hair back.

It was at least three months after Charlie came home from the hospital, that she had first shared his bed. The trailer was hard to keep warm, anyway, but that night the power was off, and snow was swirling. She had carried as many blankets as she could find, then both their coats, then all their clothes and piled them on Charlie. She shivered and looked at the bed for a minute, as if examining her work.

"I reckon you'd let me stand out here and freeze," she said, as she pulled the covers back and slipped in with him. The power came on some time during the night, but they stayed in the bed past noon. Amy came back the next night and the next, through the winter, and now into spring.

"We ain't got a baby, honey," he said again with a lot more conviction than he felt. One morning last week, she had gagged while scrambling his eggs, and he asked if she was expecting. He meant it as a joke, but she ran to the bathroom and slammed the door shut. He listened to her blow her nose and sniffle for the next half hour. "You might, but we sure ain't."

"I ain't done it with nobody else." She glared at him for a second, then her features melted in a "What's the use?" attitude that Charlie had never seen.

He leaned over and one handed his guitar into its flimsy case. He scraped ashes off the Formica tabletop and opened a new pack of cigarettes. Was she after something? He had as close to nothing as you can have…a rusted-out trailer, a couple of pairs of jeans and a bunch of T-shirts.

"This ain't no trick, Charlie," she said, like she'd read his mind.

He sucked hard on his cigarette and held the smoke deep in his lungs.

"I'm starting my third month. Doc done told me. I know it's yours because you're the only one it could be."

"What if I take a test and prove it ain't mine?"

"What kind of test is that?"

"One where they examine my piss, count the tadpoles in it or something. They's tests they can do."

"This baby ain't no tadpole, Charlie. And it wouldn't prove nuthin'," she said, "except I still got me a baby to raise."

"Well, I still ain't ready to marry," he said.

"Then you got a decision to make 'cause I won't raise my baby where it ain't wanted."

Charlie never had to wait long in Doc Corless's crowded waiting room. The receptionist always moved him to the front of the line. Charlie sat on the end of the exam table and wondered if Doc let him keep coming to break the monotony of all those old people with smelly breath waiting in the lobby.

Doc Corless burst into the room. His necktie was over his shoulder and his white coat billowed behind him like a parachute as he floated down to his stool. He held Charlie's medical folder in one hand while he searched for an ink pen with the other.

"Howareya?" Doc said before his bottom hit the stainless-steel seat.

"Alright, I reckon," Charlie said.

Doc studied him as if deciding whether he accepted "alright" as the correct answer.

When he couldn't stand the silence any longer, Charlie said, "I got me a little job at the high school." At their last appointment, Doc had encouraged Charlie to find some light work to keep him occupied until he got stronger. "It ain't official. The night janitor gives me a little money to mop for him so he can watch dirty movies in the teacher's lounge." Charlie looked to see if Doc thought that was funny.

Doc ignored him. "Amy still taking good care of you?" he asked.

Charlie hesitated and studied the floor. "She claims she's pregnant." Charlie squirmed in his chair. "Claims its mine."

Doc Corless just looked at Charlie over the top of his glasses and waited. The man was not afraid of silence.

"But it can't be. I had the mumps when I was a kid, and they fell on me."

"That doesn't always mean you're sterile," Doc said.

"I want one of them tests…"

More silence.

"That's not really the point, is it? Up until a few weeks ago, Amy cleaned your bottom. She carried you food. When has she been out of your sight?"

That was the other thing about Doc Corless. When he did decide to talk, he threw out a big net, then he hauled in the answers and filleted the biggest one on the spot. He never threw one back.

"Couldn't it mean that you've stumbled onto somebody who actually cares about you?"

Charlie limped out of the exam room. Quack army doctor, he thought. What does he know about love?

*   *   *

Charlie counted out enough cash from his last un-employment check so Amy could get through the end of the month. He tucked it in an envelope and wrote a note on the back that said he'd leave the truck parked at the bus station with the key under the floor mat. He left his guitar on the couch and considered telling her it was OK to pawn it. He thought better of it. She could make up her own mind about that. He left the trailer unlocked and headed for town.

"Where to, buddy?" the ticket agent asked.

Charlie hadn't thought about where. He remem-bered Amy and her plans to wait tables like a college kid.

"Myrtle Beach?" he asked. He didn't know if it was in North or South Carolina, so he didn't volunteer.

"The way it works is you tell me where you want to go, and I sell you a ticket," the man said.

"Myrtle Beach," Charlie said. "I wanta see the ocean." He slid a small handful of bills and change toward the man without counting it.

"That'll get you a little past Ashville."

Charlie added a smaller wad of cash to the pile. He tried to sort the money with one hand.

"What happened to your arm?"

"Vietnam," Charlie said.

The ticket man smoothed the bills and counted the change. "This'll get you there, but it won't get you back."

For the first time in months Charlie wished he had a drink. "Good," he said. "'Cause I ain't coming back."

The bus was almost empty during the ride across the Smokies. Charlie sat at the very back by the window. The moon burned high in the sky as hot as his conscience. He couldn't rid himself of his last memory of Amy standing in the doorway with her skinny shoulders hunched and her arms folded across her chest like she was trying to keep her heart from spilling out on the ground. If he was home, he and Amy would be in bed by now, his weak arm over her chest, her body curled inward on his, and her butt nestled into the bend of his waist. He could almost smell the scent of shampoo on the back of her neck.

He slept off and on, waking only when they took on passengers at stops like Knotty Branch or Swan Pond, graveled arcs in the road just wide enough to park the bus. The sun was up when they parked in the terminal at Myrtle Beach.

Charlie ate breakfast in a coffee shop before he took the short walk to the beach. The wind stood his hair up straight, then flattened it again so hard that his scalp tingled. Seagulls floated along, then stopped in midair, their forward movement exactly balanced by the wind in their face and their pounding wings. The ocean touched the skyline in the far-off distance. Rolling gray water heaved and billowed like a dirty sheet hanging on a clothesline before it flattened and rushed toward the beach. The sight of it made Charlie's stomach lift into his chest. The water stopped just at his feet, paused, then ran back the way it came. It seemed to huddle out on the horizon to gather its strength and roar at him again.

He noticed a woman not much older than Amy sitting on a beach towel watching her toddler play in the sand. He tottered to his mom who pulled him to her lap and hugged him. The baby giggled and looked toward Charlie, a half-eaten cheerio in his hand, his nose running and sand crusting on his face.

Charlie wanted to tell her about Amy, but instead he said, "Babies are a handful, ain't they?"

Mom wiped the baby's nose so hard that the little guy twisted his head away, grimaced and cried for ten seconds before he was grinning again. She looked exhausted. "He's worth it," she said.

Charlie smiled as he waded out to meet the waves. Something squished under his foot. He slipped, staggered, then found his balance again by waving his good arm around. He bent to examine the place where he had just stepped. The tide had retreated once more leaving nothing but a cup full of ocean trapped in his footprint. He stood in the moist sand and waited for the water to return and spill over his feet. He listened to the roar of the ocean, the baby's laughter, the sound of his heart beating faster and faster.

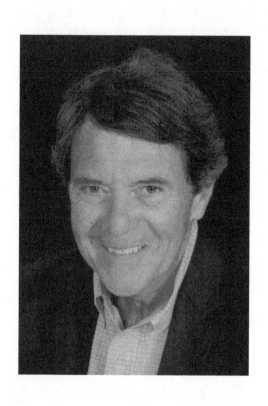

ABOUT THE AUTHOR

Ron Lands grew up in a small East Tennessee town with a five generation Appalachian pedigree containing a host of farmers and preachers, but no writers or physicians. As he states, "The first indication that I might break that mold was the day after President Kennedy's assassination when, in an attempt to process that tragedy, I wrote a very bad poem and gave it to my second-grade teacher. The teasing I endured from my peers after she read it to my class squelched any desire to share work for the next twenty-five years."

His earliest interest in the medical profession occurred a year later after he developed appendicitis. As he recalls, "A small-town general practitioner performed emergency surgery late one night without a specialist's consultation, abdominal CT scan or anything else considered standard today. I was enchanted by the whole process, the doctor who visited me at random times, the nurse who changed my bandage daily, and cleaned my fingertips with alcohol so I could feel the thick silk sutures."

Over five decades later, now a retired cancer doctor in Knoxville, Tennessee, he confides how he was drawn to that specialty because "the art of medicine has remained relevant even as the science has unfolded in breathtaking waves." He still works part-time because he enjoys learning new things from his young, smart colleagues, and he still enjoys clinical medicine. "I still find myself writing to find clarity about my patients. Writing and medicine are my vocation and avocation, impossible to do one without the other."

He lives and writes near his hometown, still married to the nursing student he met while in medical school. He is the proud father of a son and daughter, and delighted father-in-law to the mother of his two granddaughters.

He is an MFA alumnus of Queens University of Charlotte. His short stories have been published in several small literary journals. His clinical vignettes and poems have been published in the humanities sections of medical journals. His first chapbook, *Final Path*, was published in the spring of 2020. A second poetry collection, *A Gathering of Friends*, is forthcoming in the fall of 2021.

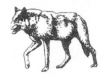

BOOKS BY BOTTOM DOG PRESS
HARMONY SERIES

The Pears: Poems, by Larry Smith, 66 pgs, $15
Without a Plea, by Jeff Gundy, 96 pgs, $16
Taking a Walk in My Animal Hat, by Charlene Fix, 90 pgs, $16
Earnest Occupations, by Richard Hague, 200 pgs, $18
Pieces: A Composite Novel, by Mary Ann McGuigan, 250 pgs, $18
Crows in the Jukebox: Poems, by Mike James, 106 pgs, $16
Portrait of the Artist as a Bingo Worker: A Memoir,
by Lori Jakiela, 216 pgs, $18
The Thick of Thin: A Memoir, by Larry Smith, 238 pgs, $18
Cold Air Return: A Novel, by Patrick Lawrence O'Keeffe, 390 pgs, $20
Flesh and Stones: A Memoir, by Jan Shoemaker, 176 pgs, $18
Waiting to Begin: A Memoir, by Patricia O'Donnell, 166 pgs, $18
And Waking: Poems, by Kevin Casey, 80 pgs, $16
Both Shoes Off: Poems, by Jeanne Bryner, 112 pgs, $16
Abandoned Homeland: Poems, by Jeff Gundy, 96 pgs, $16
Stolen Child: A Novel, by Suzanne Kelly, 338 pgs, $18
The Canary: A Novel, by Michael Loyd Gray, 196 pgs, $18
On the Flyleaf: Poems, by Herbert Woodward Martin, 106 pgs, $16
The Harmonist at Nightfall: Poems of Indiana, by Shari Wagner, 114 pgs, $16
Painting Bridges: A Novel, by Patricia Averbach, 234 pgs, $18
Ariadne & Other Poems, by Ingrid Swanberg, 120 pgs, $16
The Search for the Reason Why: New and Selected Poems,
by Tom Kryss, 192 pgs, $16
Kenneth Patchen: Rebel Poet in America, by Larry Smith,
Revised 2nd Edition, 326 pgs, Cloth $28
Selected Correspondence of Kenneth Patchen,
Edited with introduction by Allen Frost, Paper $18/ Cloth $28
Awash with Roses: Collected Love Poems of Kenneth Patchen,
Eds. Laura Smith and Larry Smith
with introduction by Larry Smith, 200 pgs, $16
Breathing the West: Great Basin Poems, by Liane Ellison Norman, 96 pgs, $16
Maggot: A Novel, by Robert Flanagan, 262 pgs, $18
American Poet: A Novel, by Jeff Vande Zande, 200 pgs, $18
The Way-Back Room: Memoir of a Detroit Childhood,
by Mary Minock, 216 pgs, $18

BOTTOM DOG PRESS, INC.

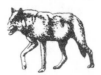

P.O. BOX 425 /HURON, OHIO 44839
HTTP://SMITHDOCS.NET